Diseases desperate grown
By desperate appliance are relieved
Or not at all

Hamlet, Act 4, Scene 3

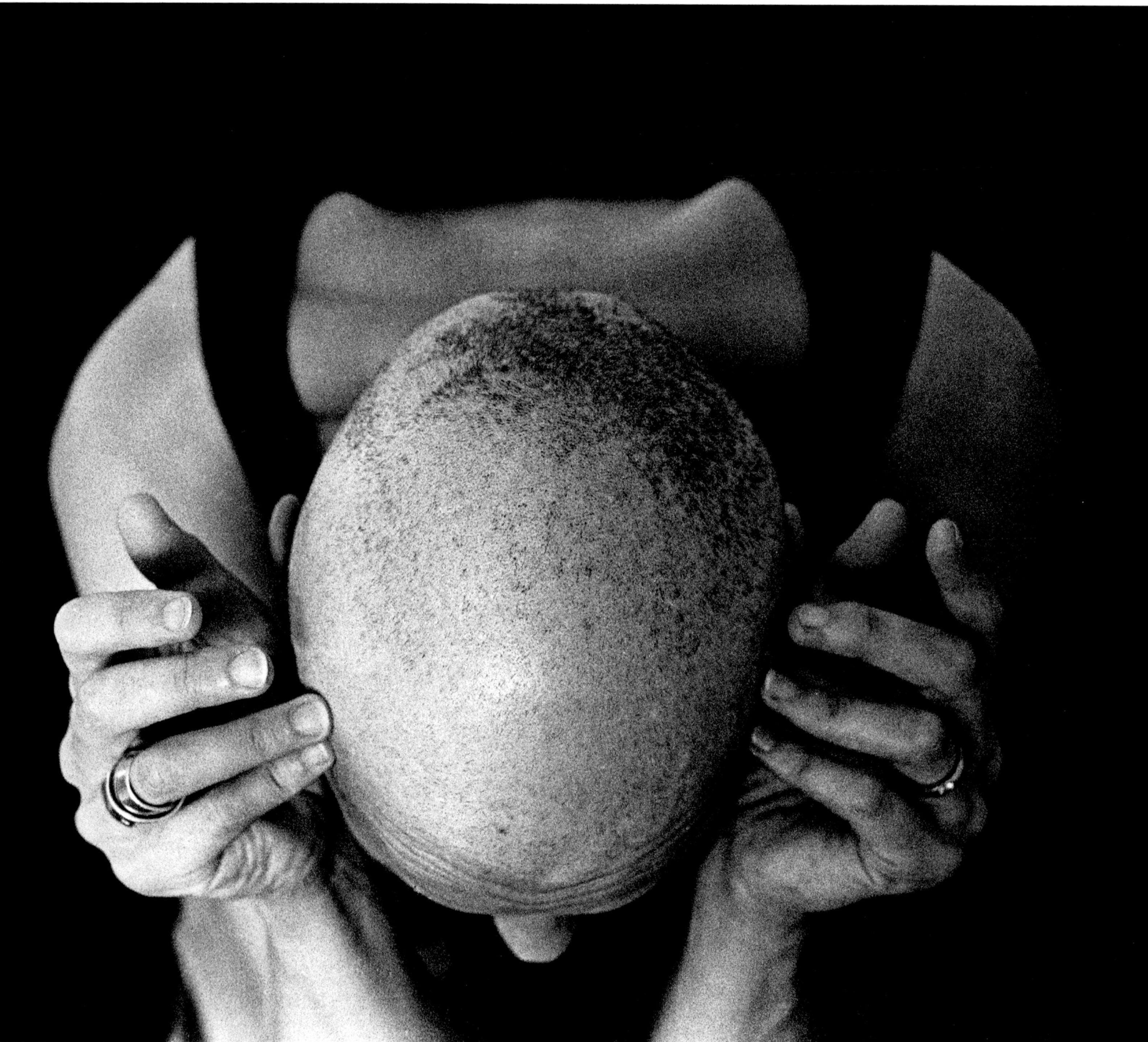

BEYOND FEAR

CAROLINE SEYMOUR

DEWI LEWIS PUBLISHING

These photographs were taken over the last five years. The subject, broadly, is cancer; the desperate disease that calls for such desperate appliances as surgery, chemo- and radiotherapies. Many of them were taken in operating theatres, of surgeons at work on patients. Hands move in pools of light, cutting, holding, stitching, swabbing; appearing white against the blackness like the hands of mime artists. Their gestures and the creased folds in the surgeons' sleeves like those in Renaissance and later paintings, the patients wrapped and draped like pietàs. A perfectly sculptural body, subjected to disease and medical intervention, wears its imperfections like the ageing of ancient marbles. And the theatre we are in has its own drama and intensity: a theatre of flesh, bone, steel and light.

I was fortunate to be given access to this hidden world. Hidden, that is, to the patients themselves, who are always unconscious there, and inaccessible to anyone who is not a medic. The photographs show several different procedures: post-mastectomy breast reconstructions using the patient's own tissue, an eye-shaped 'flap' cut from their abdomen by plastic surgeons, and the removal of rare and aggressive bone cancers called sarcomas, by orthopaedic surgeons.

Caroline Seymour

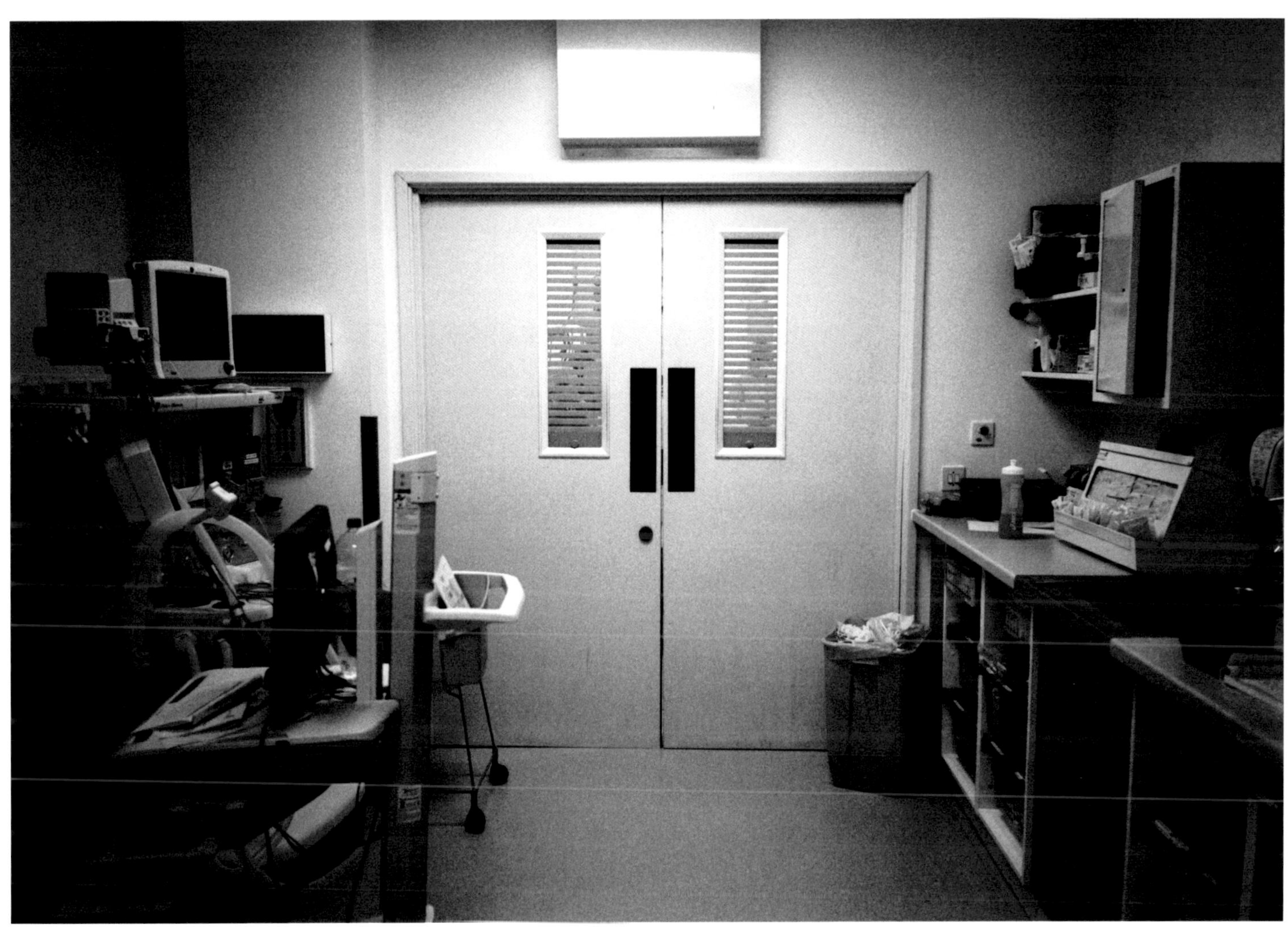

Morbidity and mortality are obscured within our society. Naturally, both present themselves eventually for us all, but when they do, we often encounter them in hospitals, hospices, or hidden in our homes, or as horrors in films and stories, in which we might see the image of a decomposing body, or bear witness to mortal wounds inflicted violently, or discover someone has locked away infirm relations in an attic. Many of us shudder at the idea of an open casket funeral, opting instead for a closed coffin, that will be slid slowly by conveyer belt to be cremated behind a curtain.

In the life story of the historical Buddha, Siddhartha Gautama, it was prophesied at his birth that he would become either a powerful king or a religious leader. His father, a clan chieftain himself, believed that shielding his son from the reality of old age, sickness and death, would lead him to fulfill his worldly rather than spiritual destiny. When Siddhartha finally leaves the home in which he has been forcefully cocooned, he meets an old man, a sick man, and a dead man. It is through this contact with reality that he is driven to seek a deeper understanding of himself, the human condition, and the world.

This fragility, the ephemerality of everything we encounter, simultaneously induces fear and inspires, confronting us with the fact we are alive now and will not always be. It has the capacity to provoke the pursuit of meaning, and to find beauty within the pain of transience.

The people who have given permission to include photographs of their surgeries in this book demonstrate admirable bravery and generosity. The aesthetics of Caroline Seymour's work transmute this vulnerability into images that present the viewer with an honest yet humane window, rather than a voyeuristic or clinical perspective. We paint everything in the colours of our imagination and find deeper meaning through the meeting of the unavoidable reality of things and the inherent poetic nature of the human mind. These photographs capture and express moments that confront and soothe, infusing procedures on the edge of life and death with humanity and meaning.

James Ginzburg

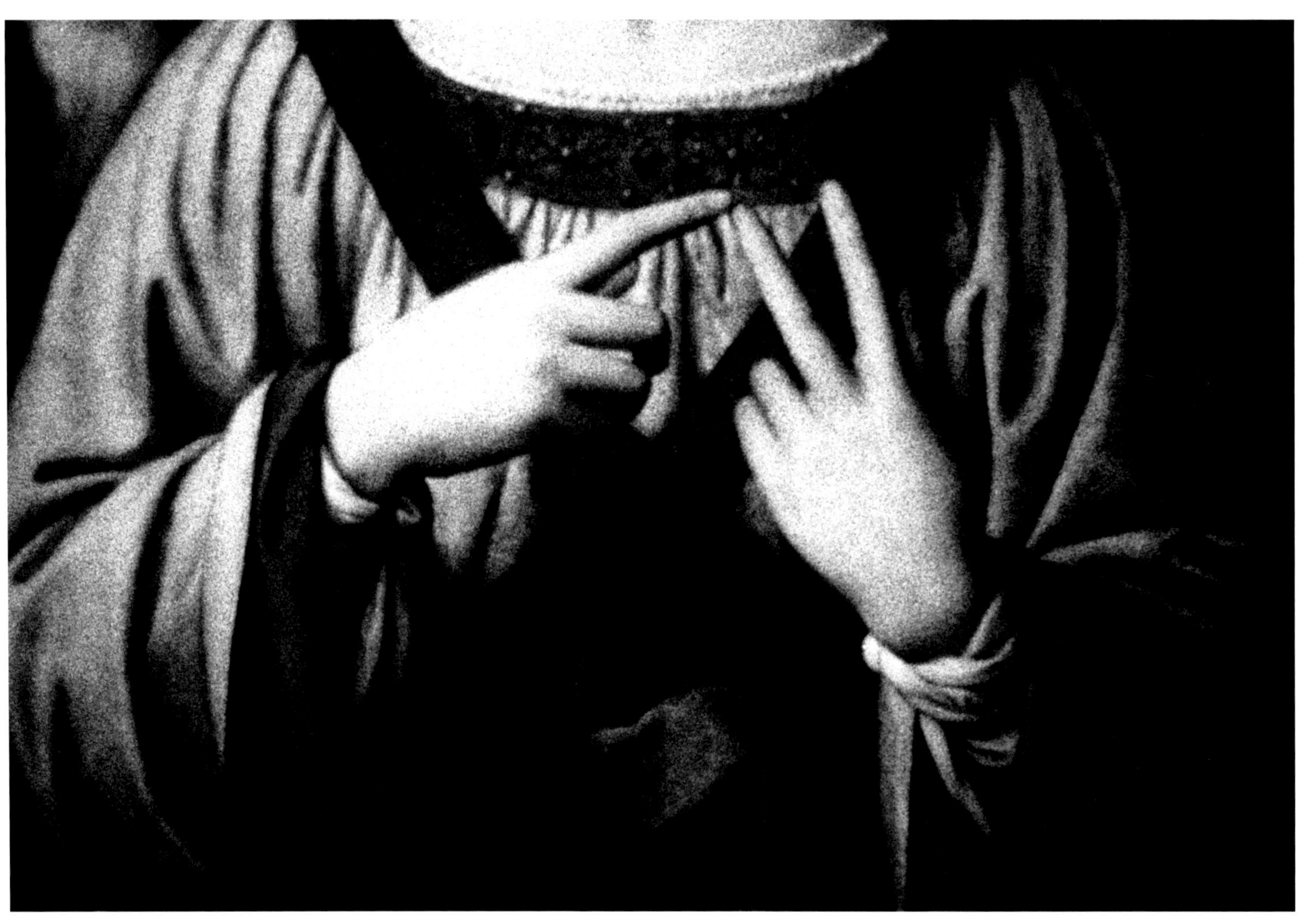

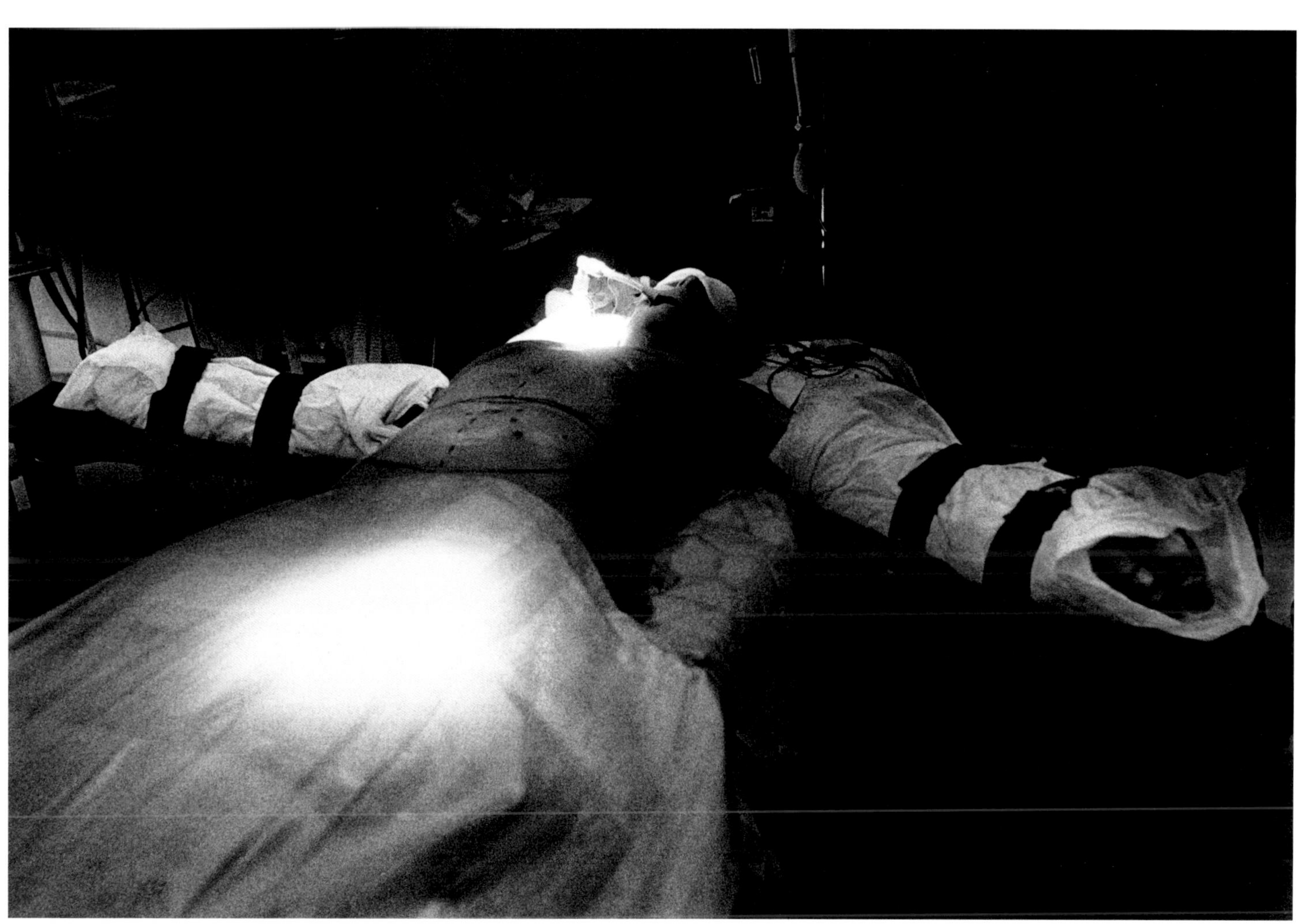

The day before surgery. A doctor herself and therefore knowing what was about to happen, she has drawn arrows pointing towards the tumours in the left breast and lymph nodes and dotted lines where the surgeon will cut. She invited me to touch. I could feel the unnatural hardness of diseased tissue beneath the skin.

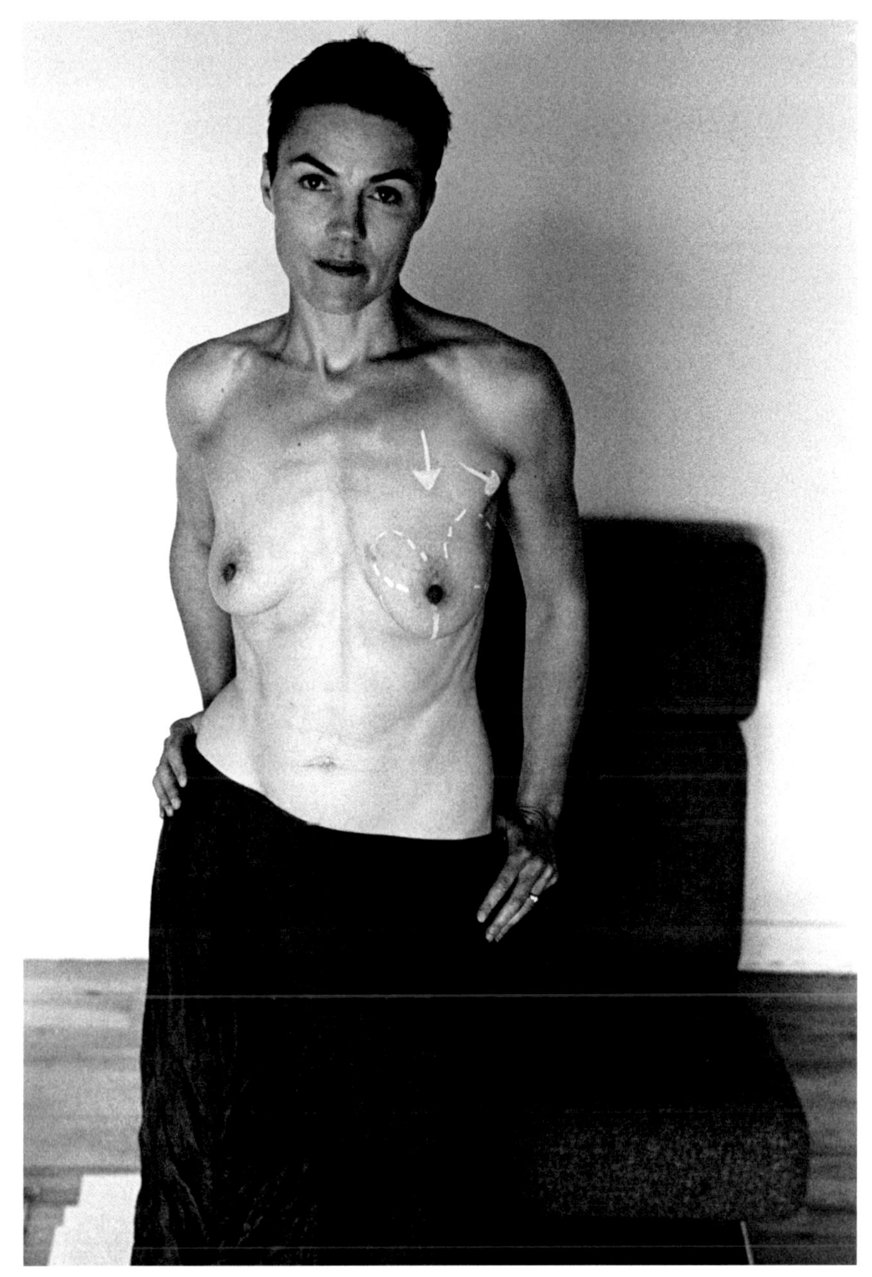

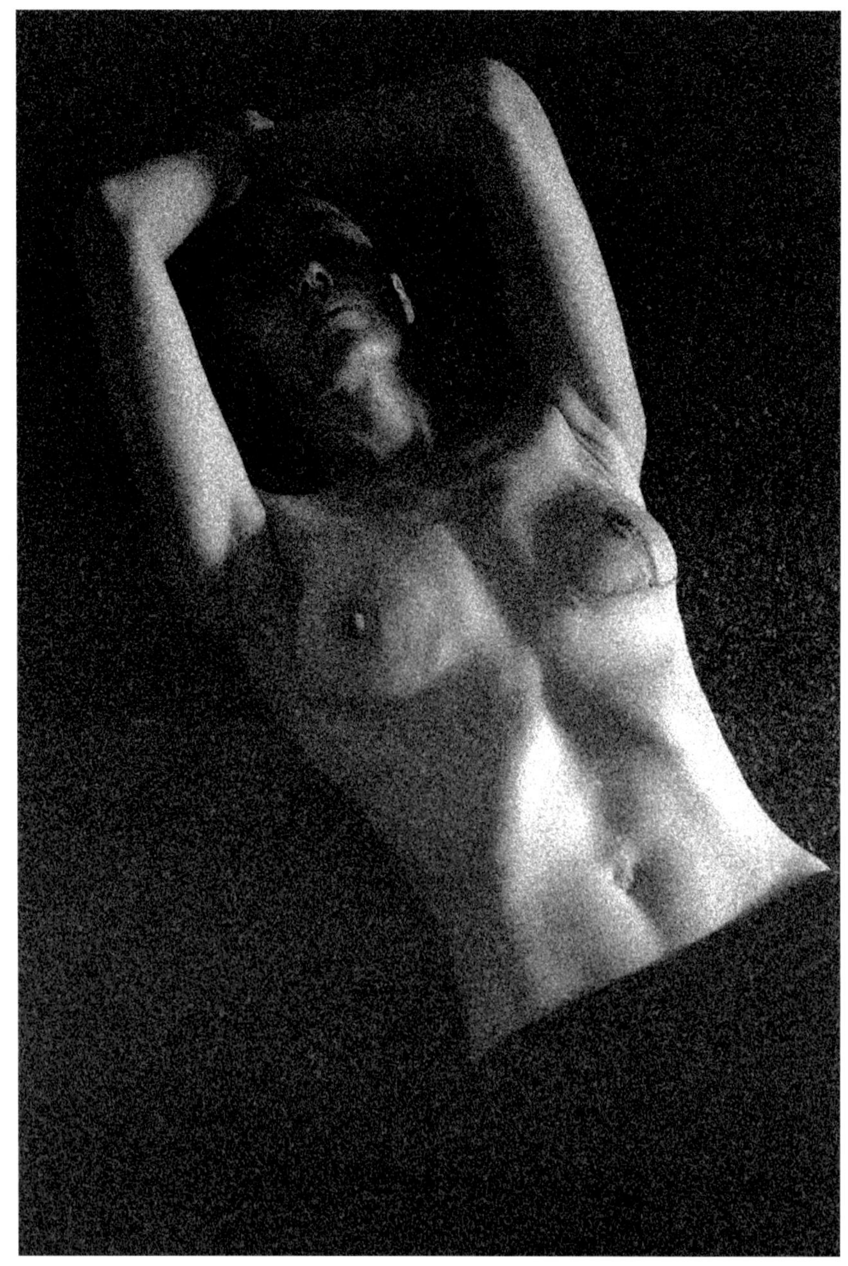

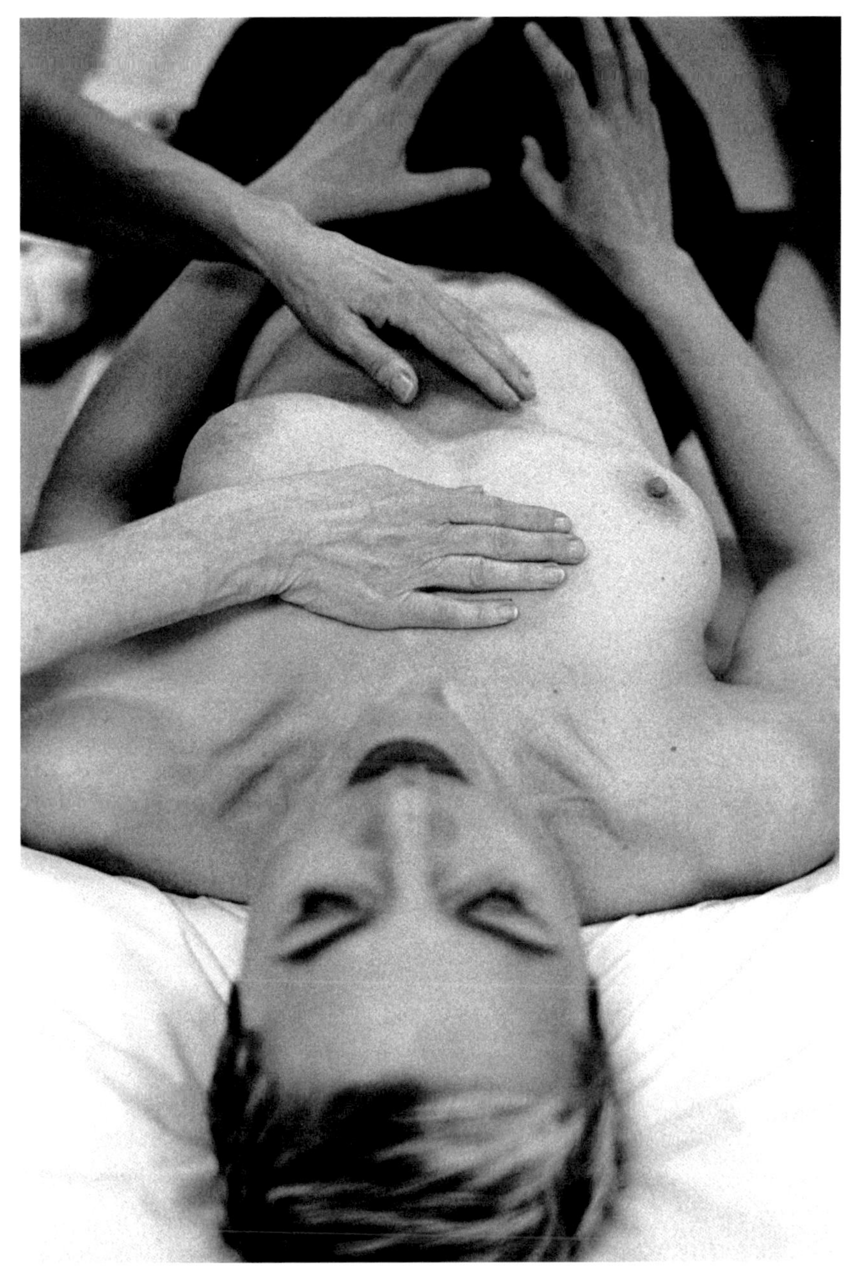

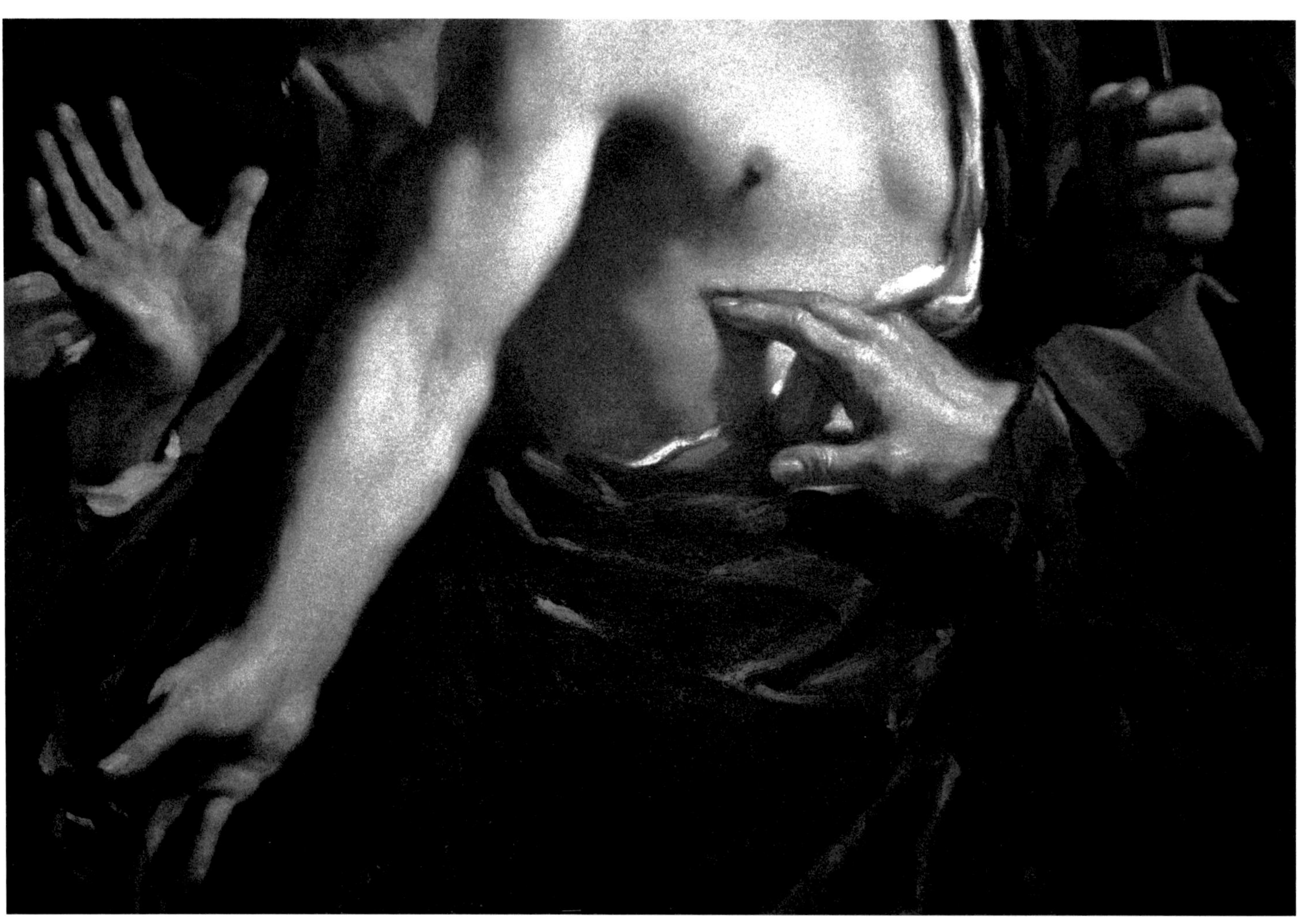

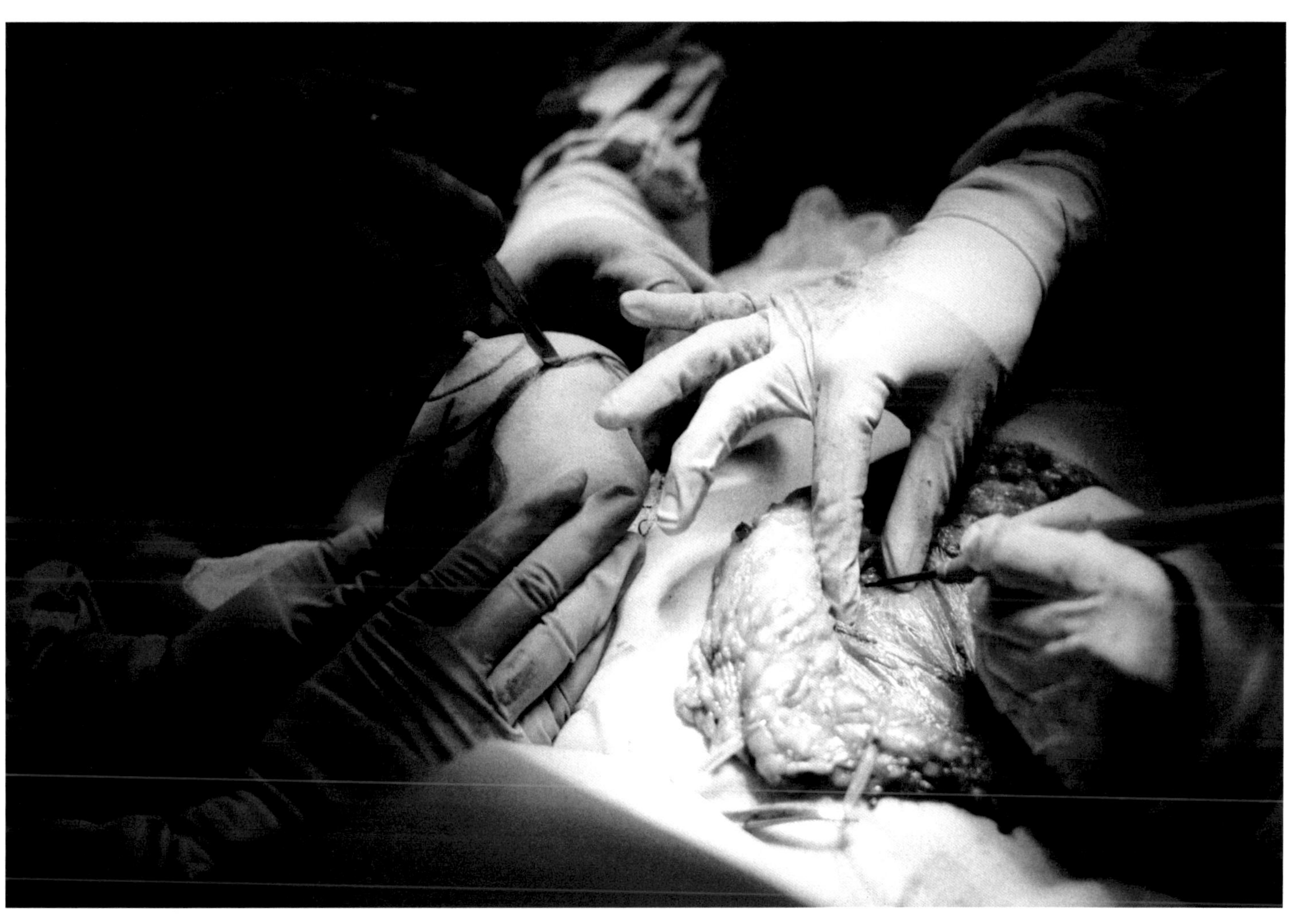

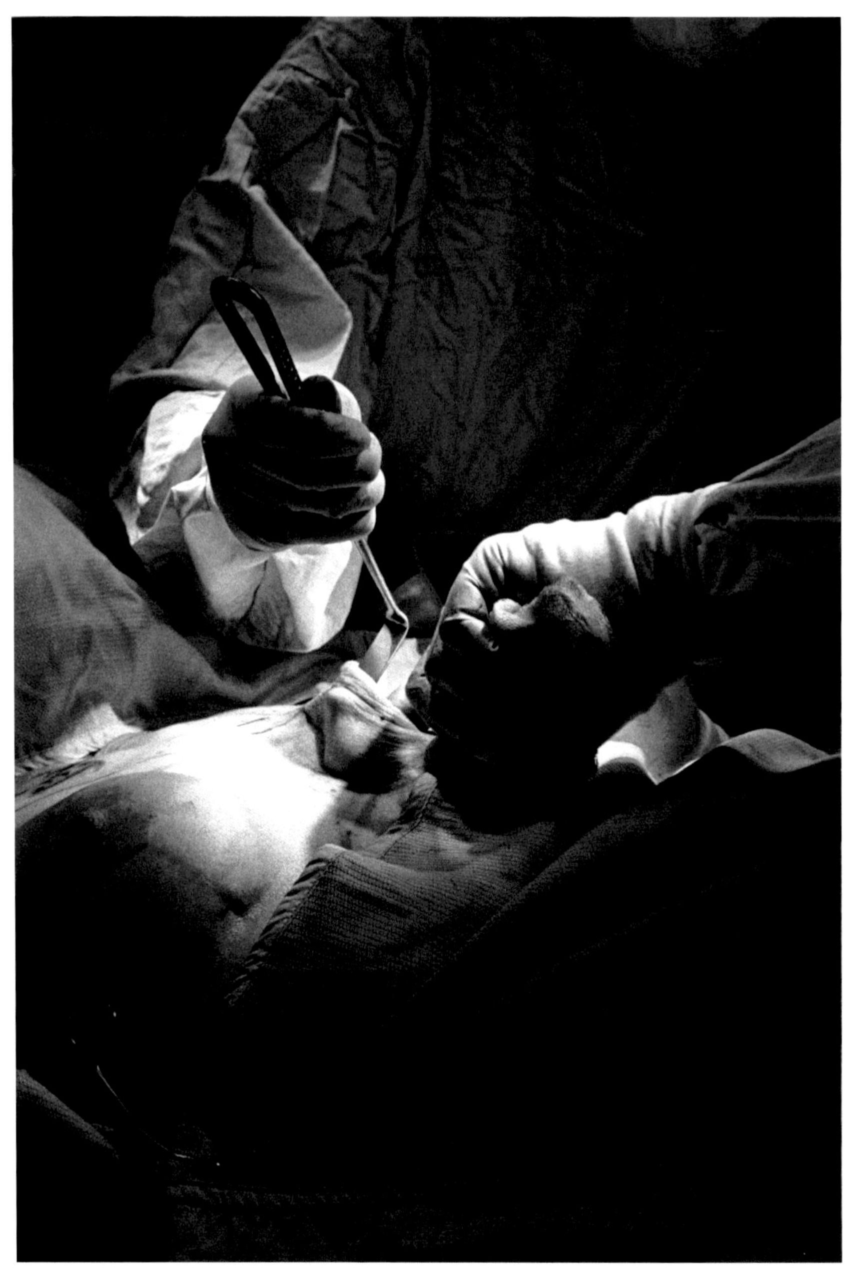

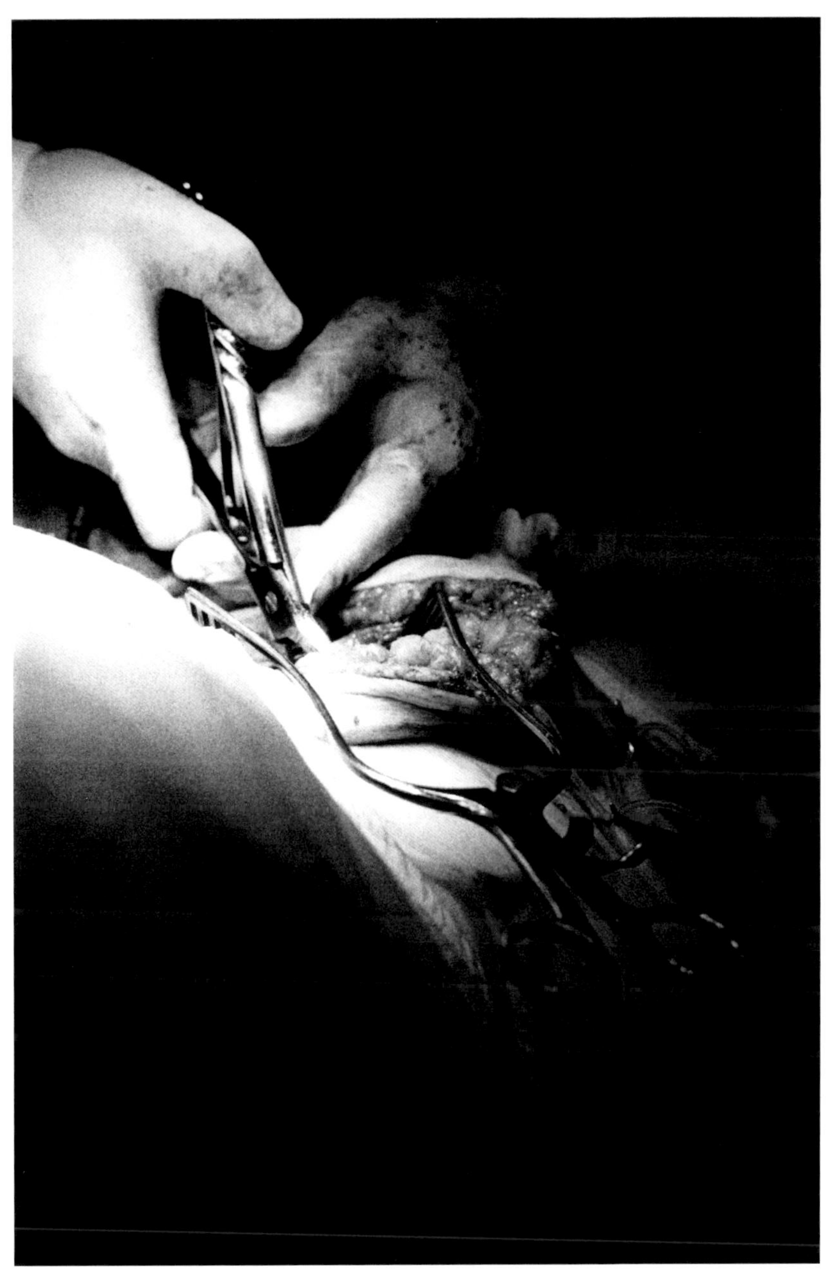

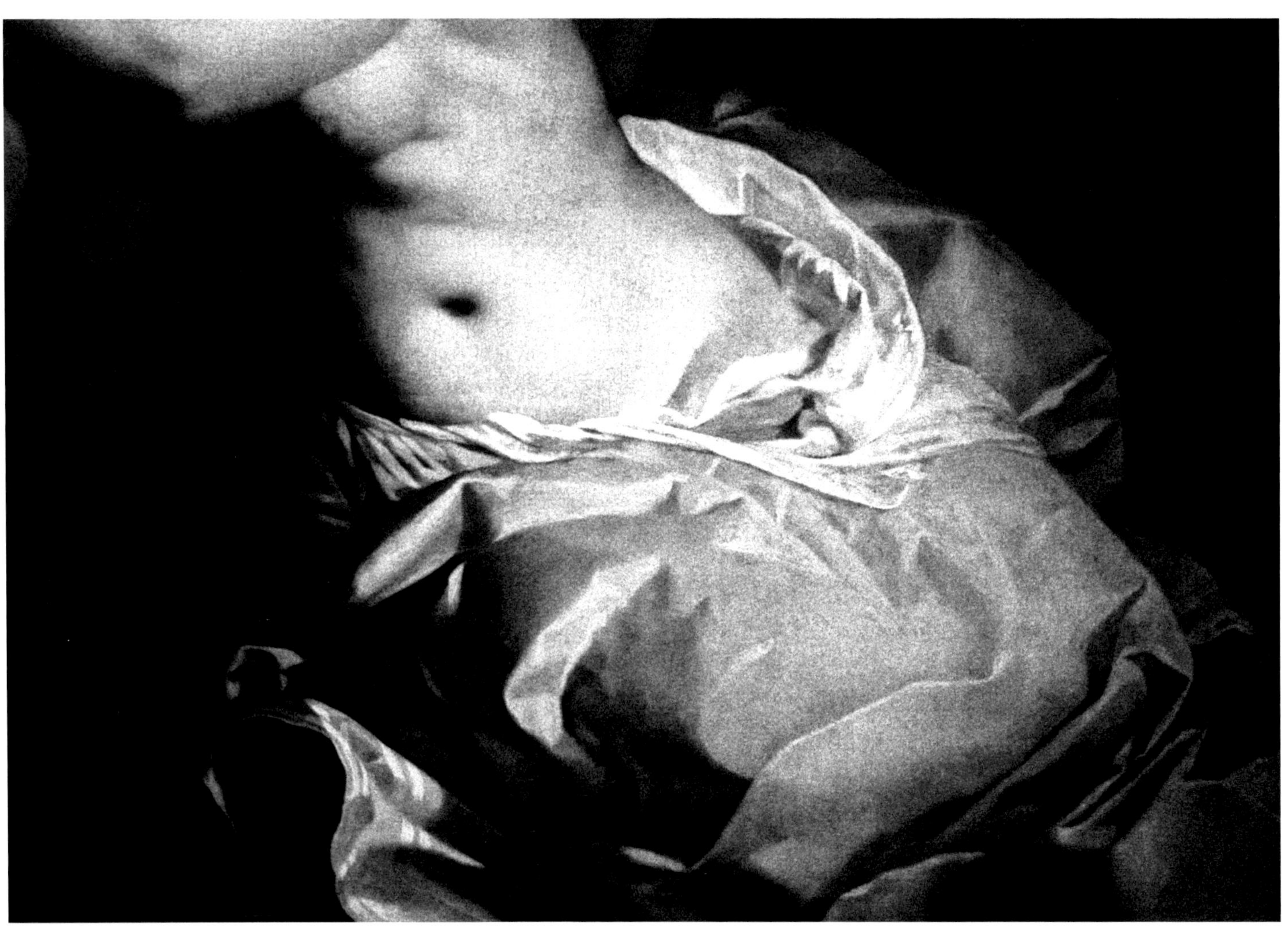

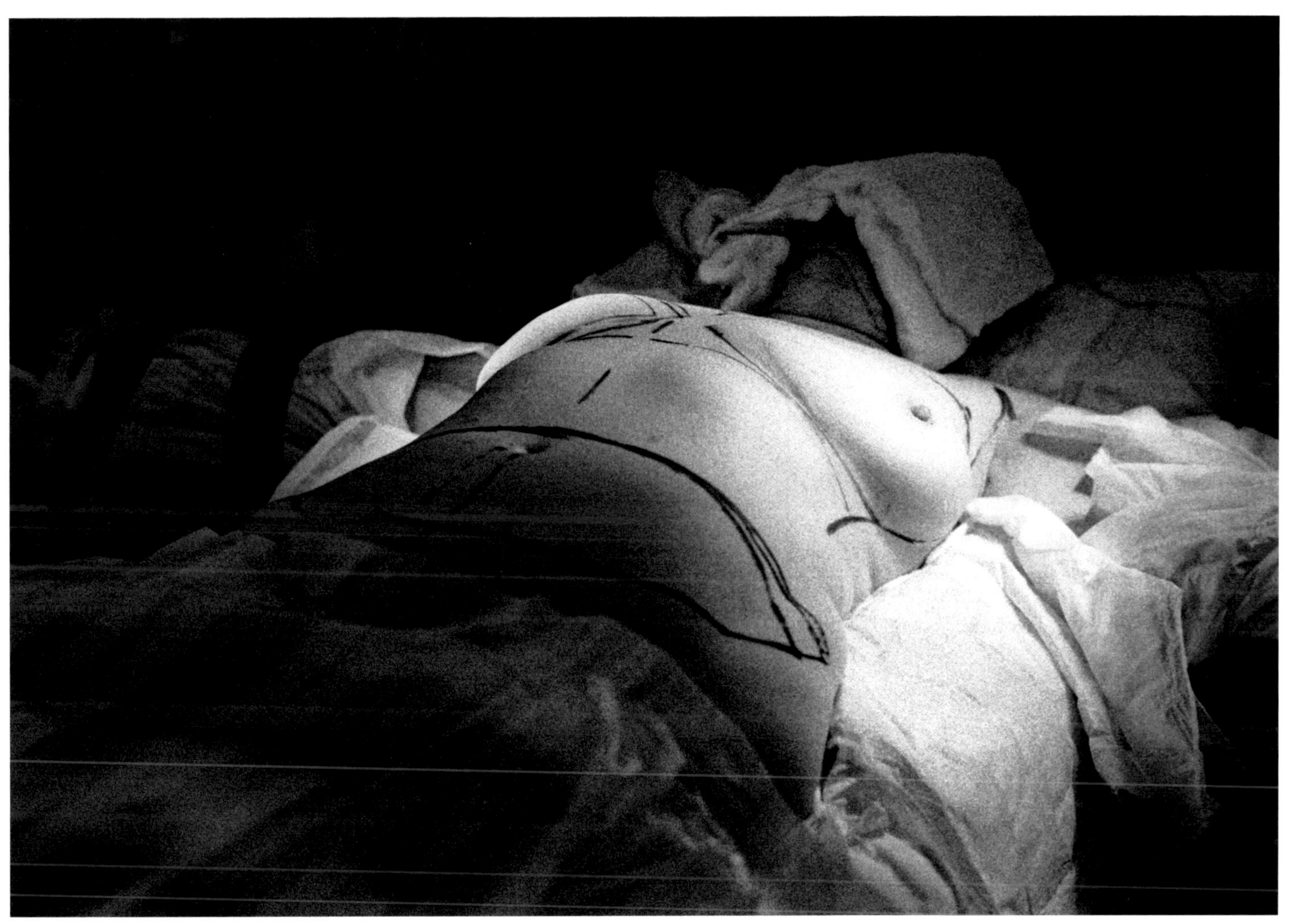

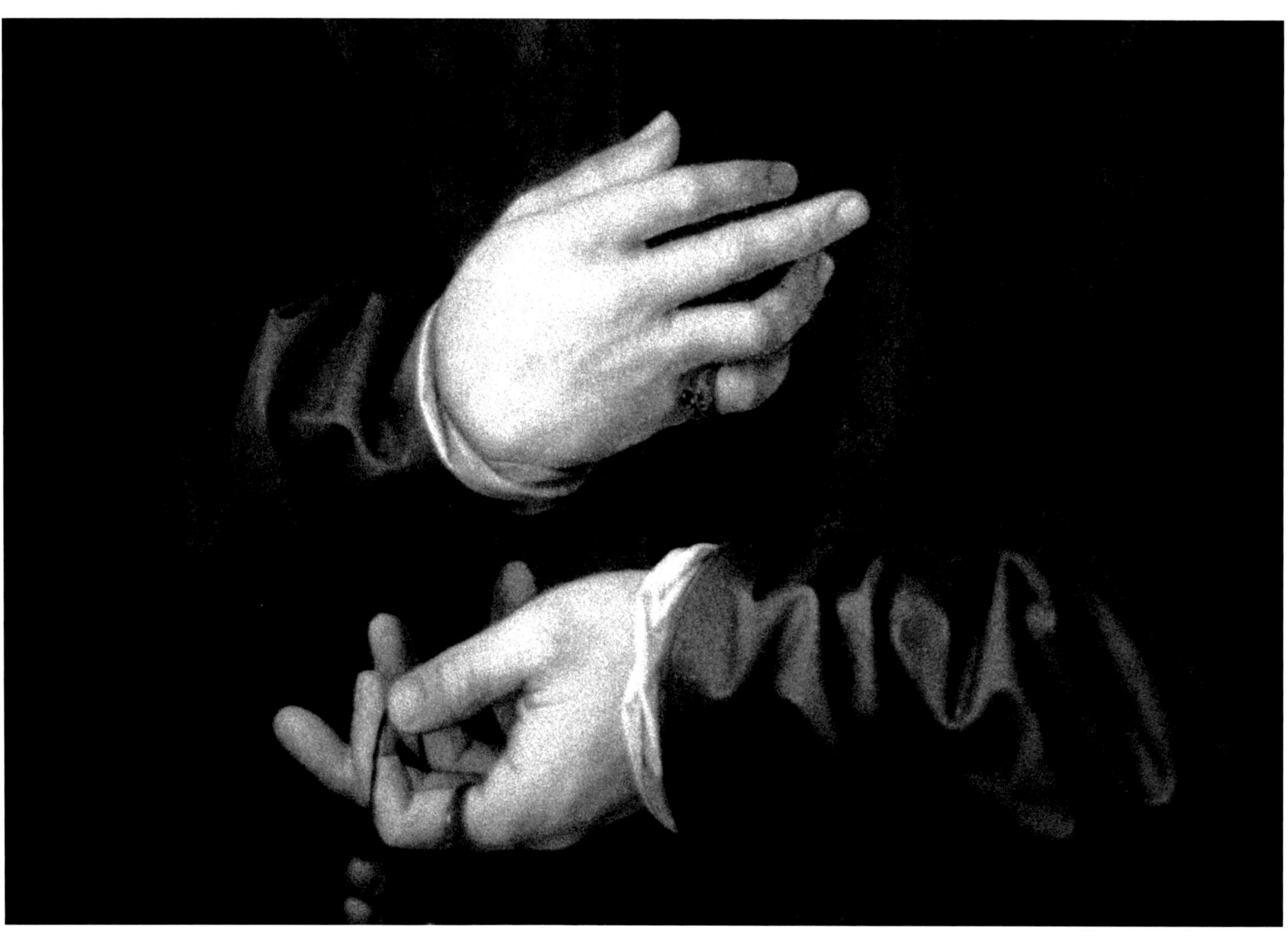

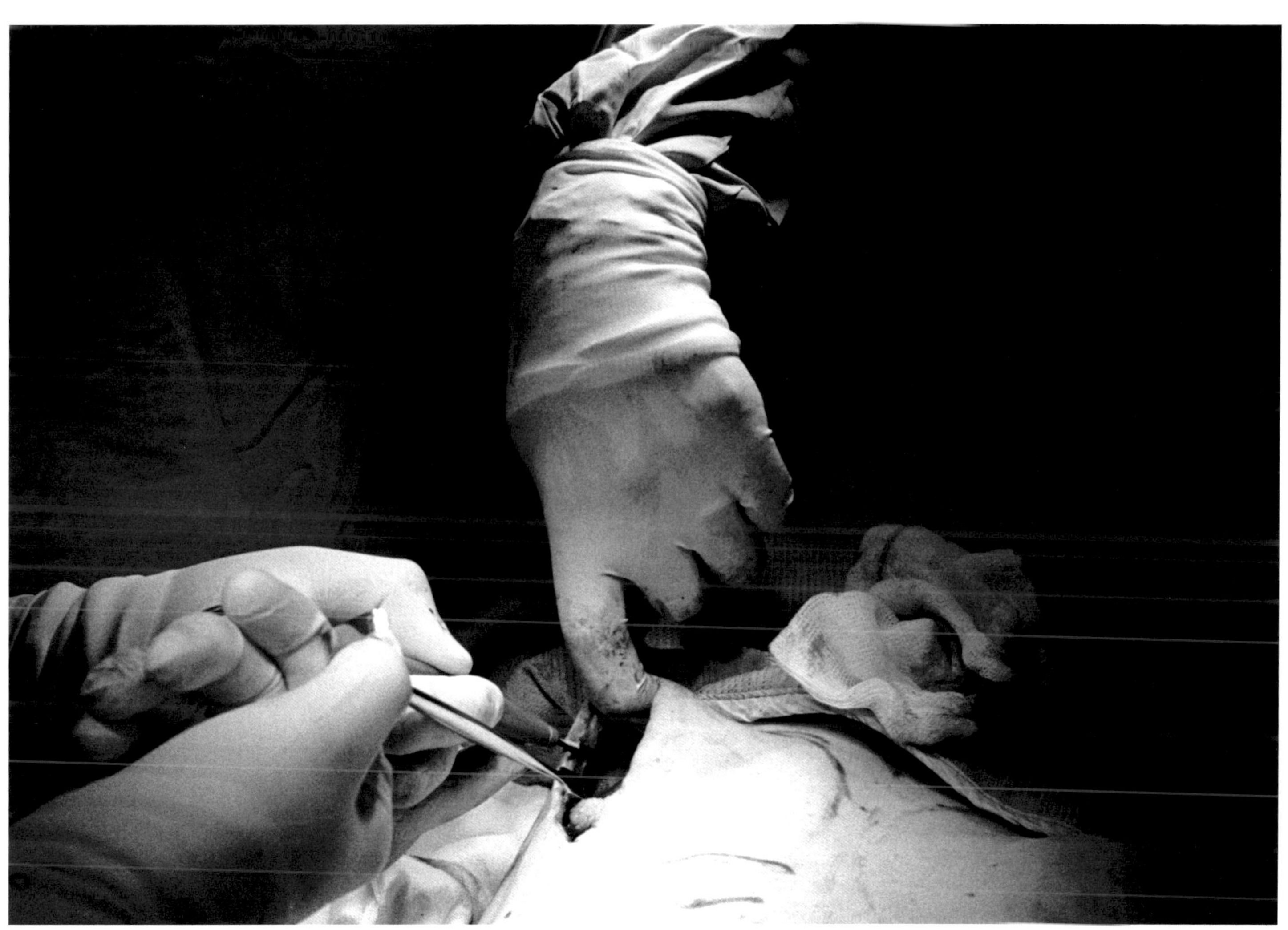

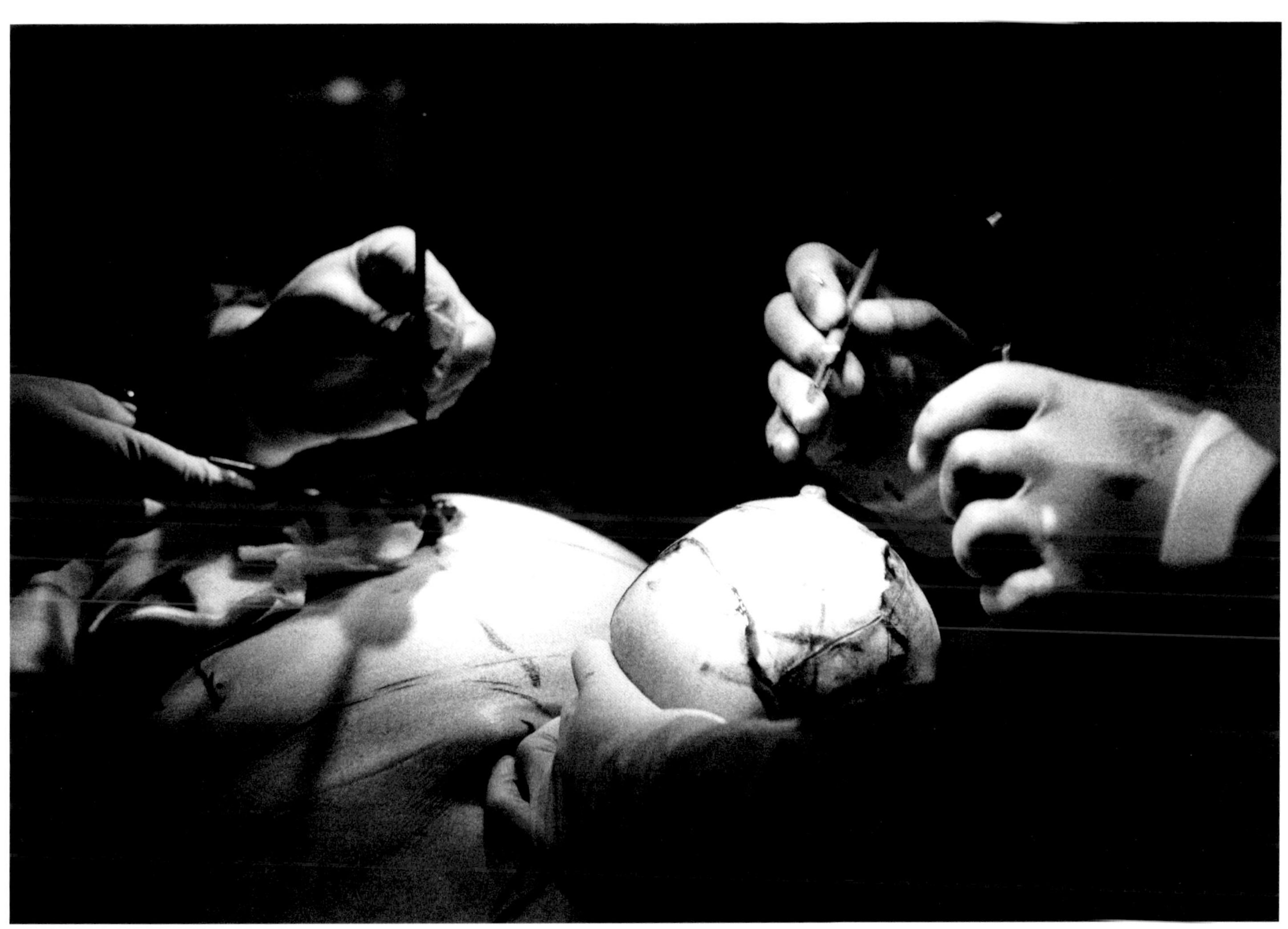

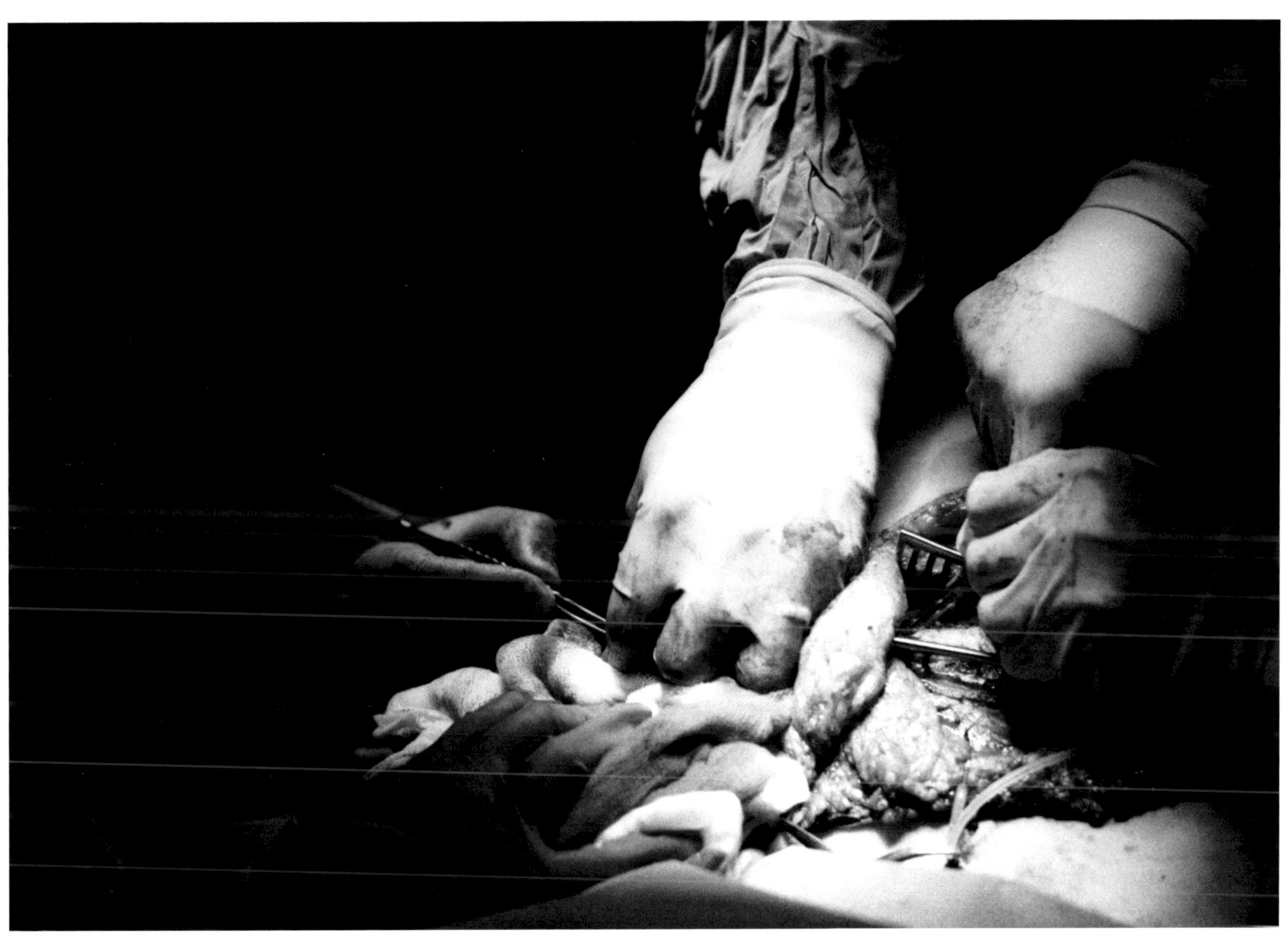

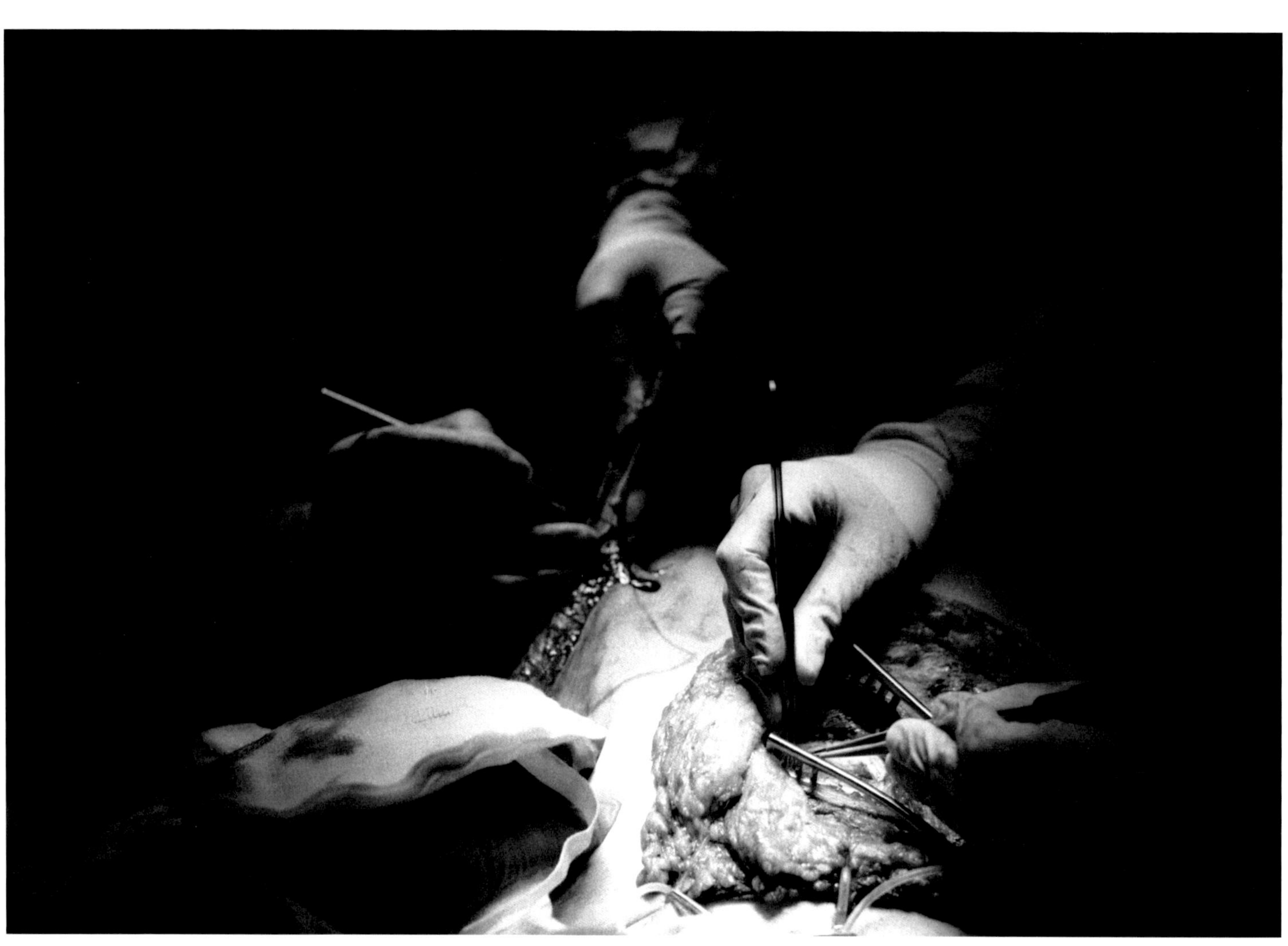

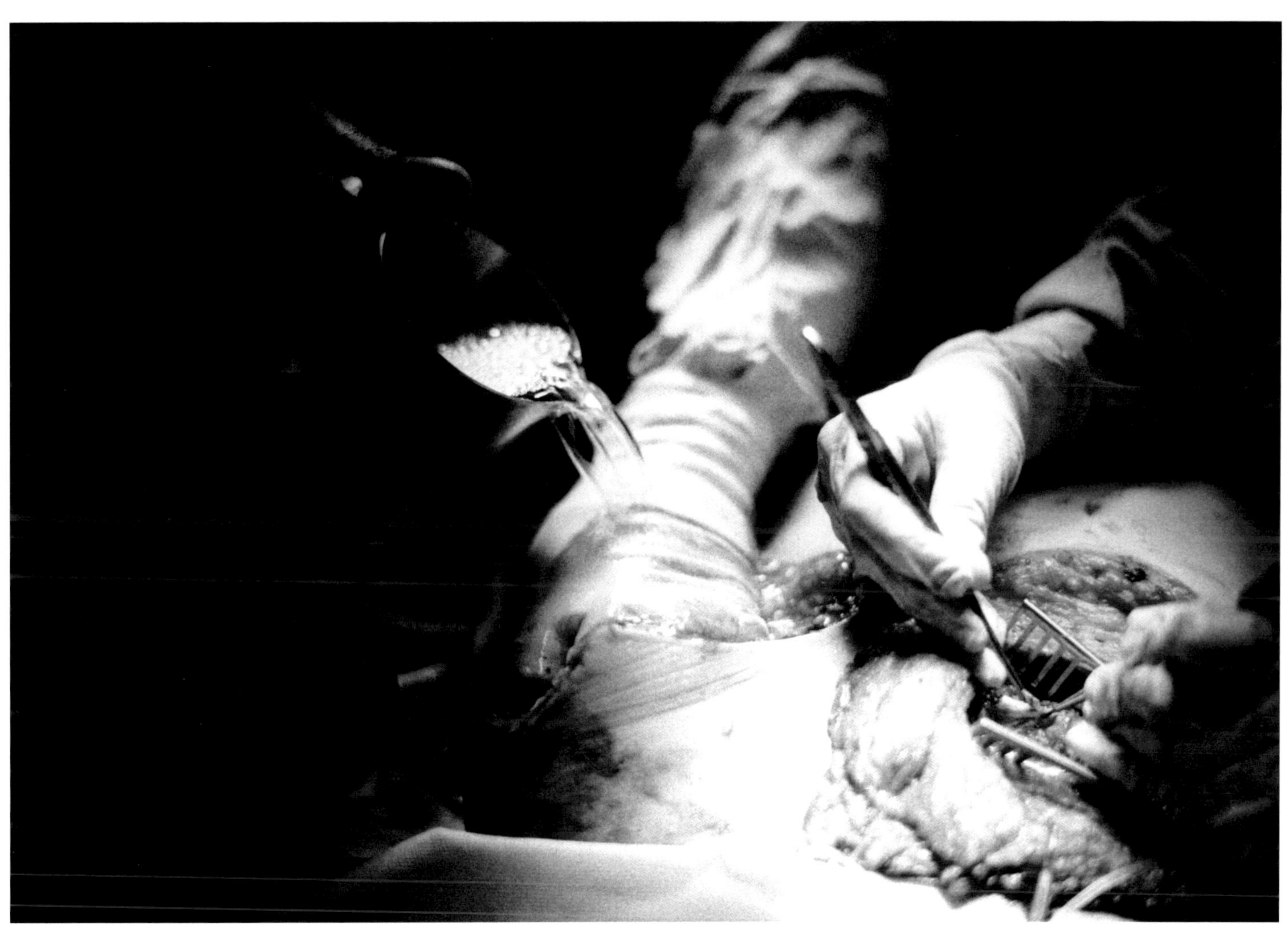

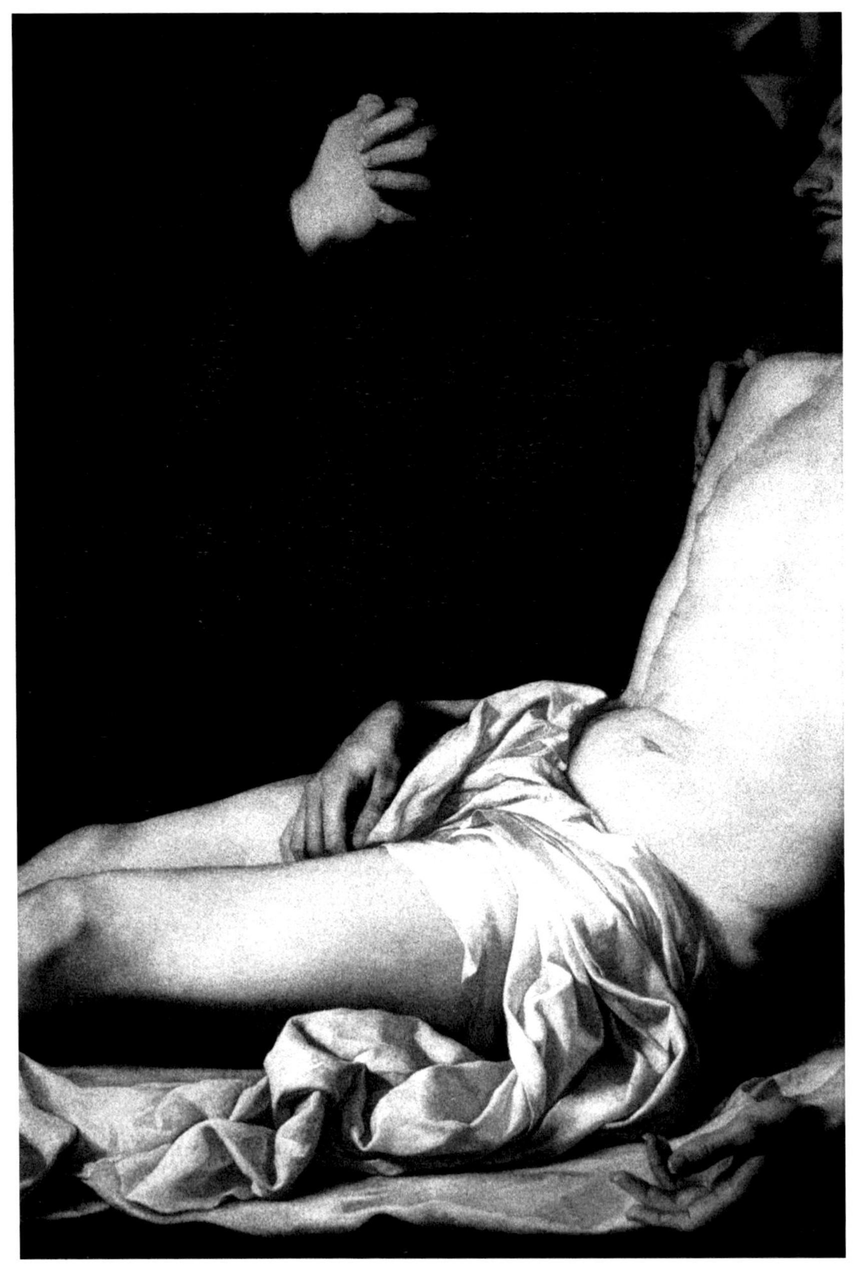

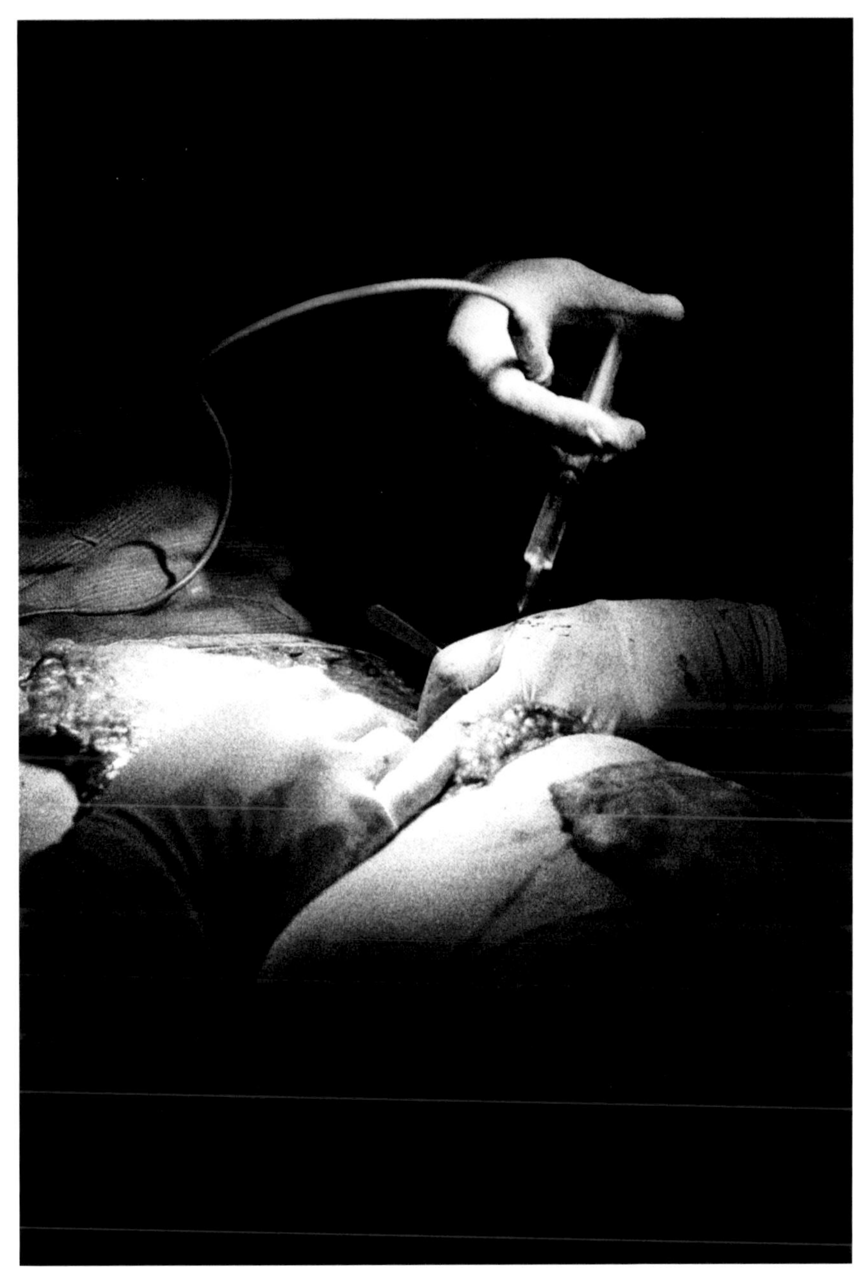

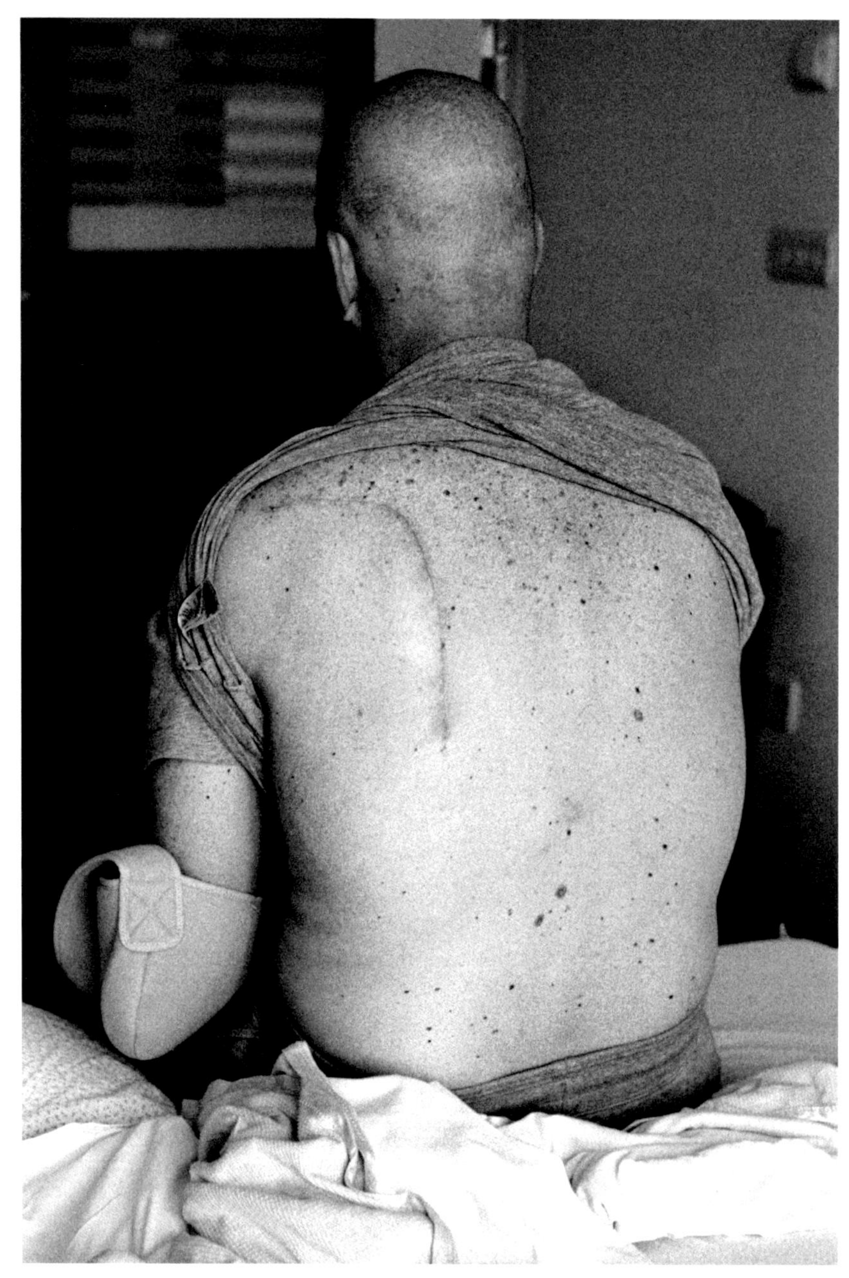

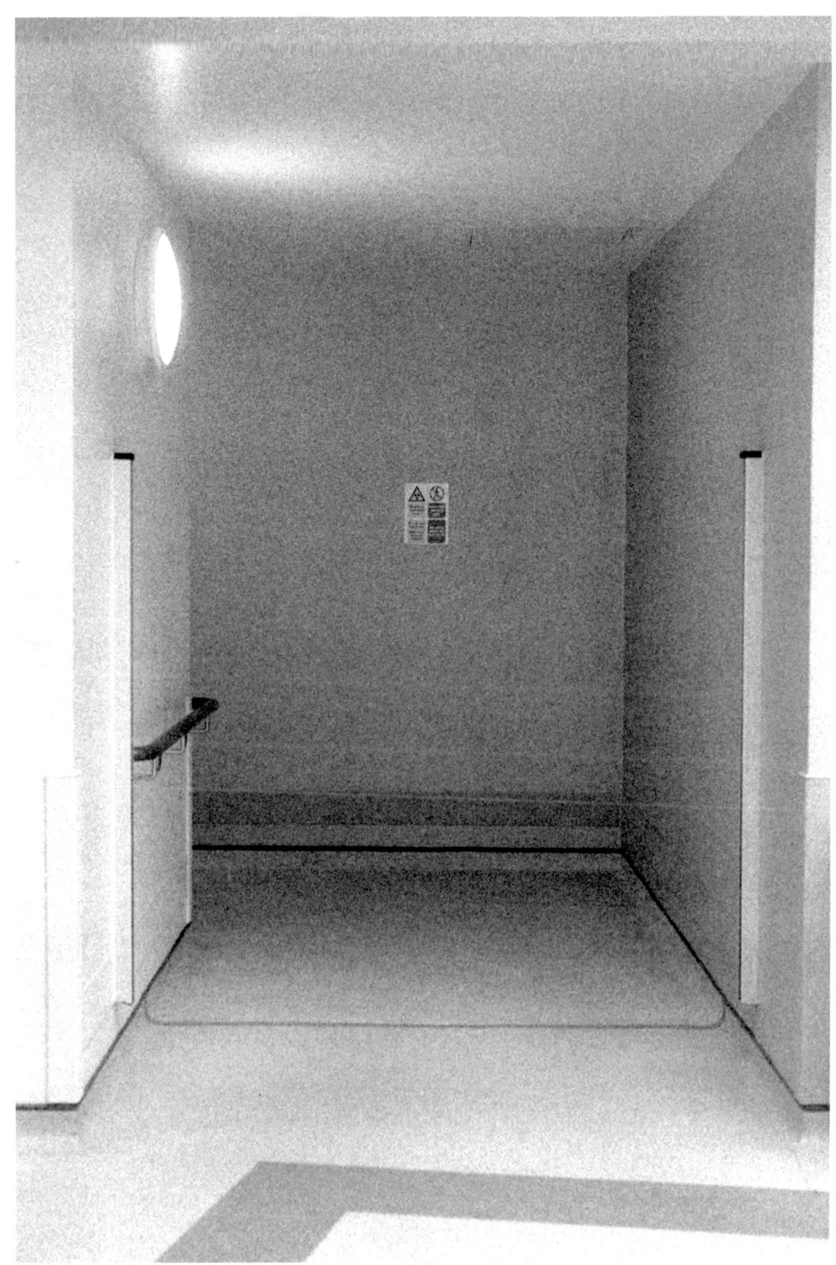

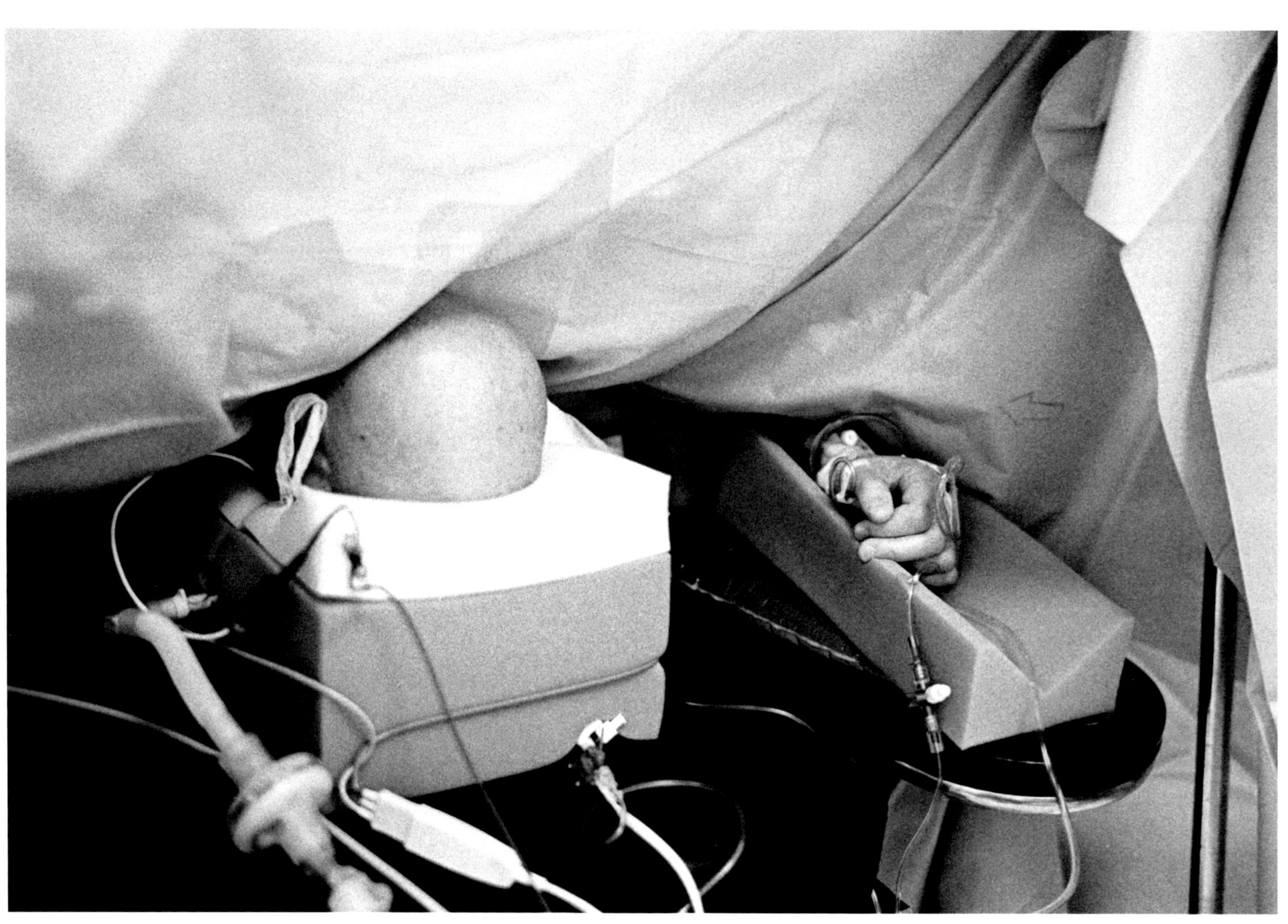

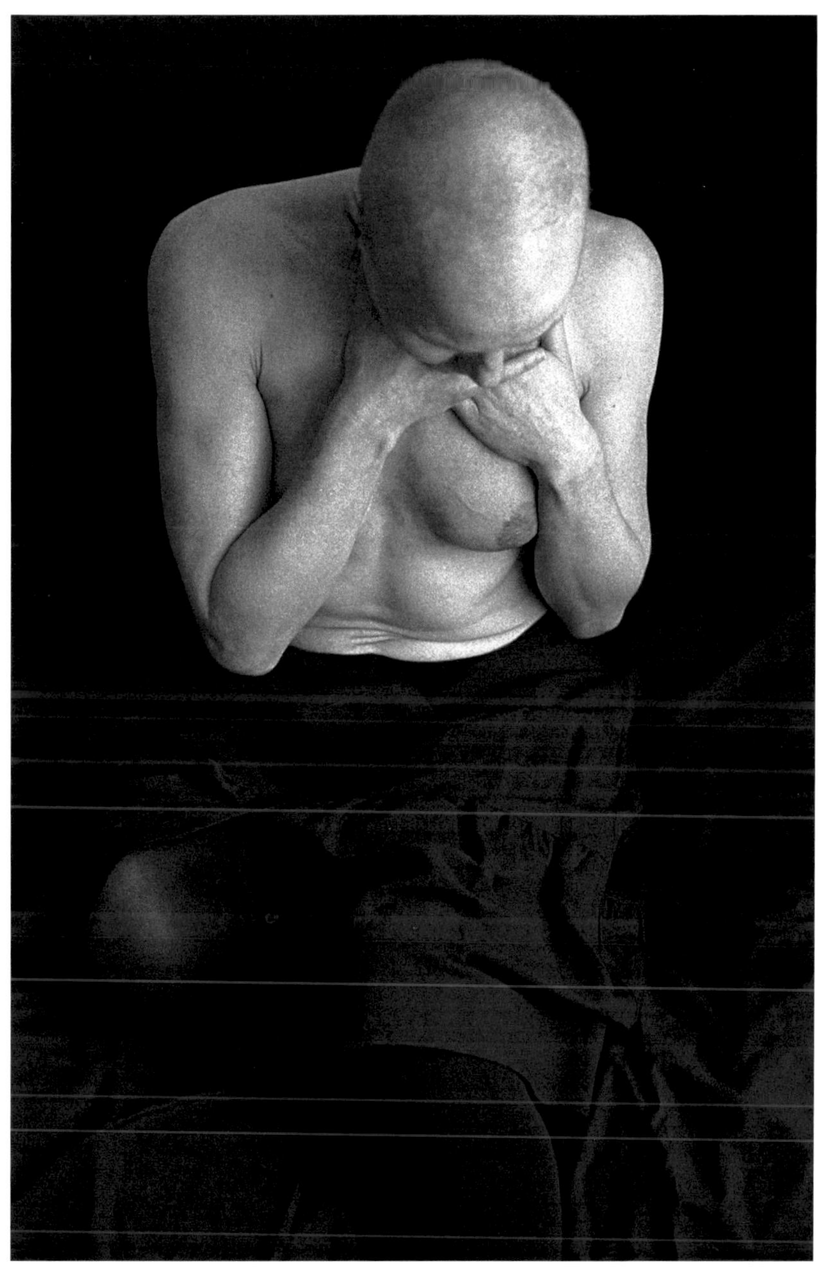

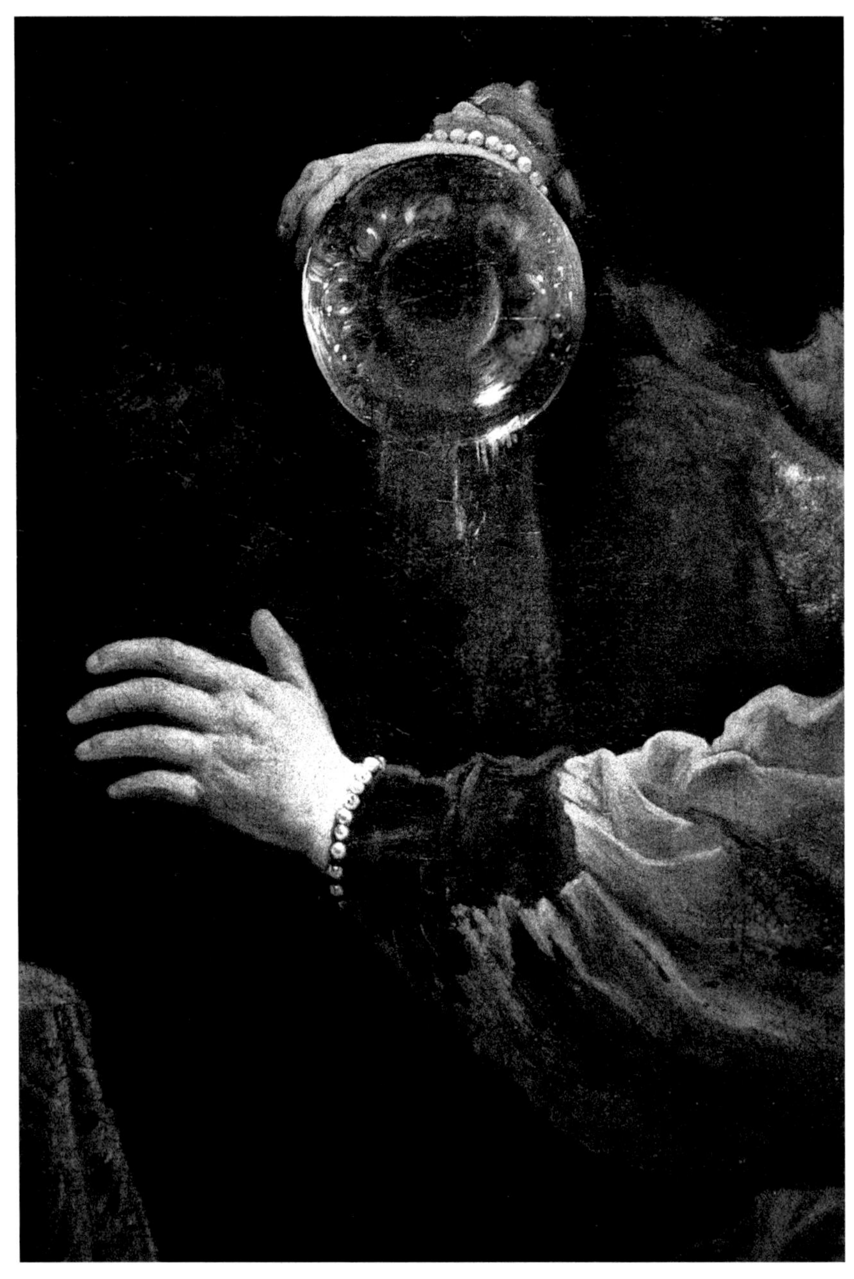

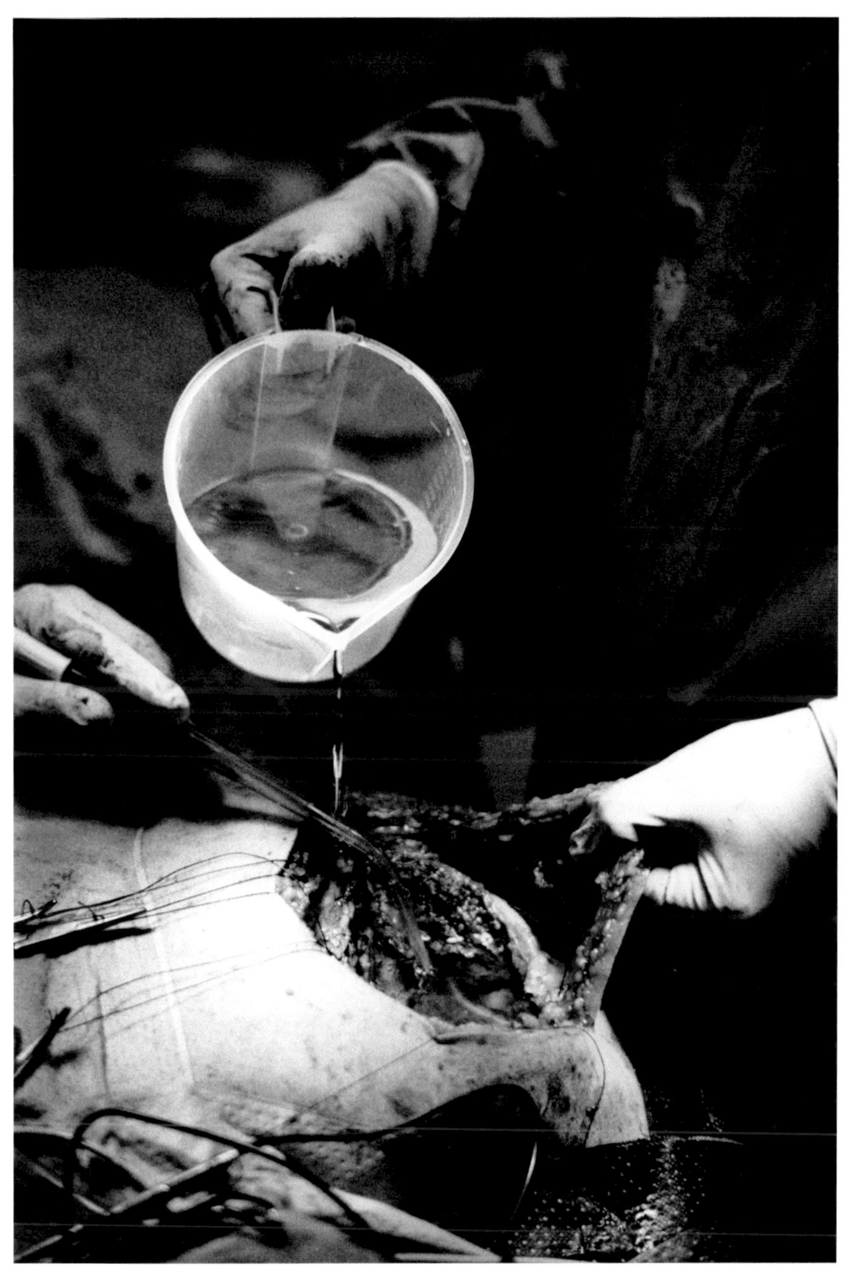

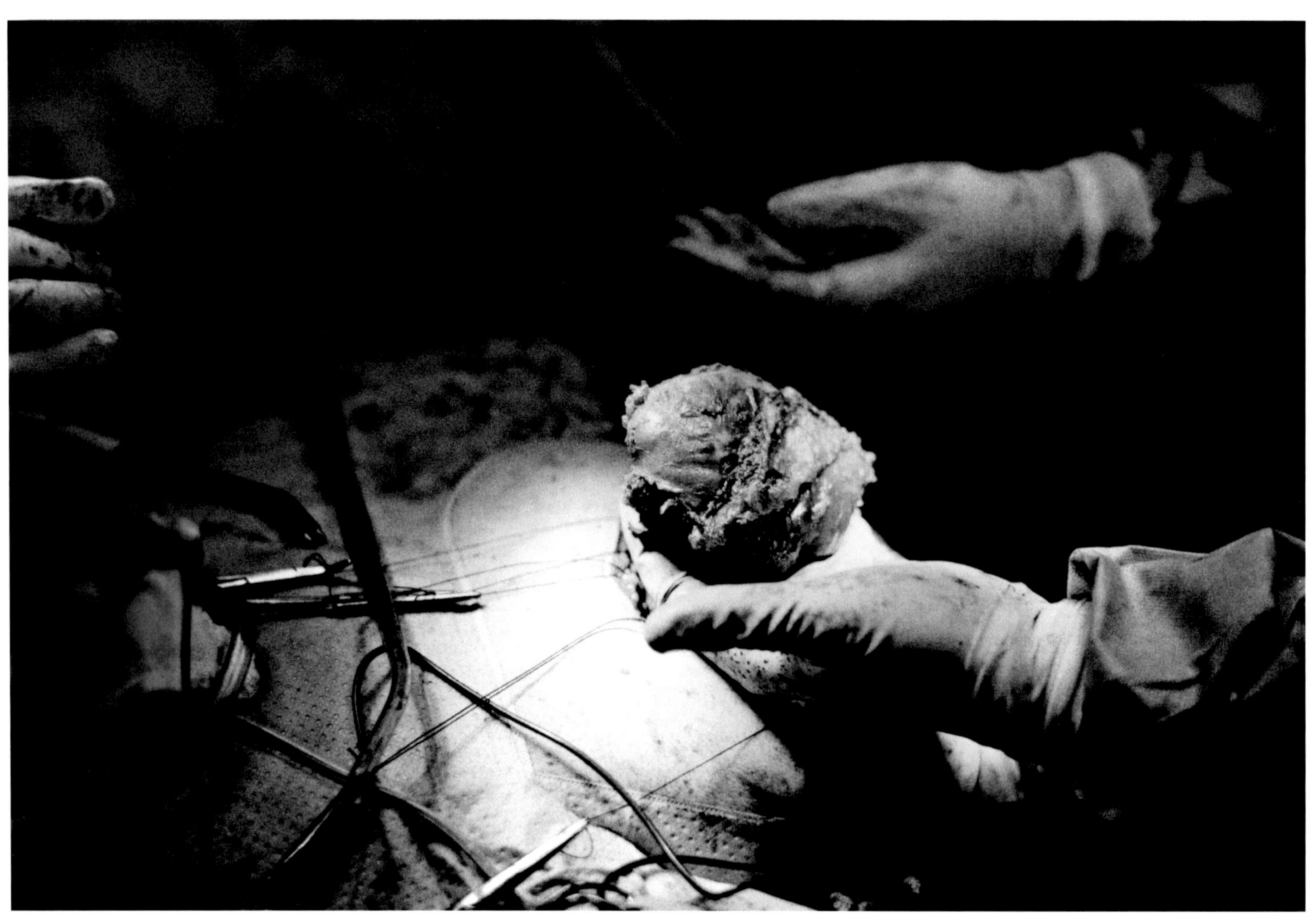

"I used to swim three or four times a week and did a lot of sport as well. I thought at first that maybe I'd just pulled a muscle or trapped a nerve. But in Hungary my mother noticed a big ball on my left scapula, within a day.

That was the first sign. It grew overnight.

The Ewing sarcoma usually affects young people. It's a very rare bone cancer. I think only a couple of dozen people a year are diagnosed with it, and since I'm forty-three this year I'm right at the outer limit of the age range. People often lose limbs with this condition."

Here is his tumour, there he is with his left arm raised, in the position of front crawl, which he will never be able to do again.

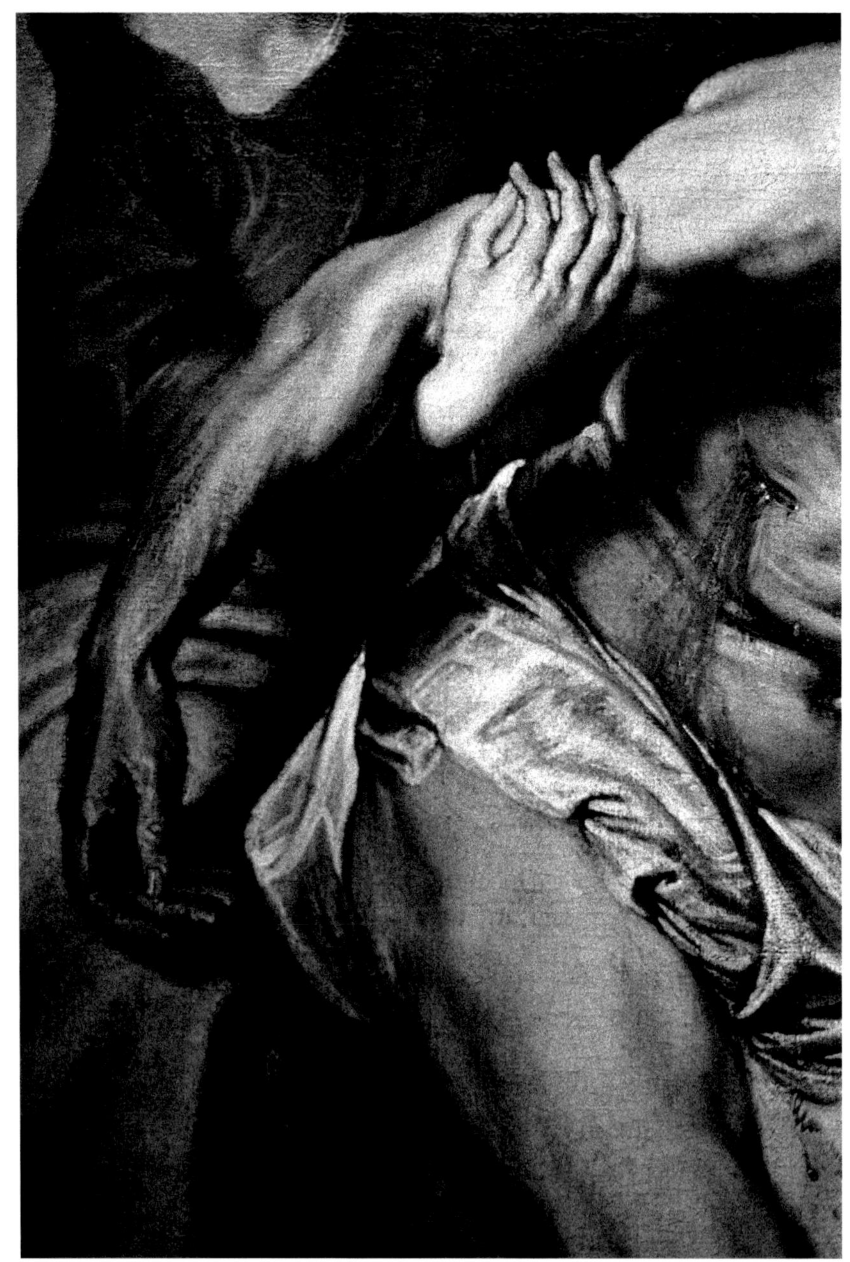

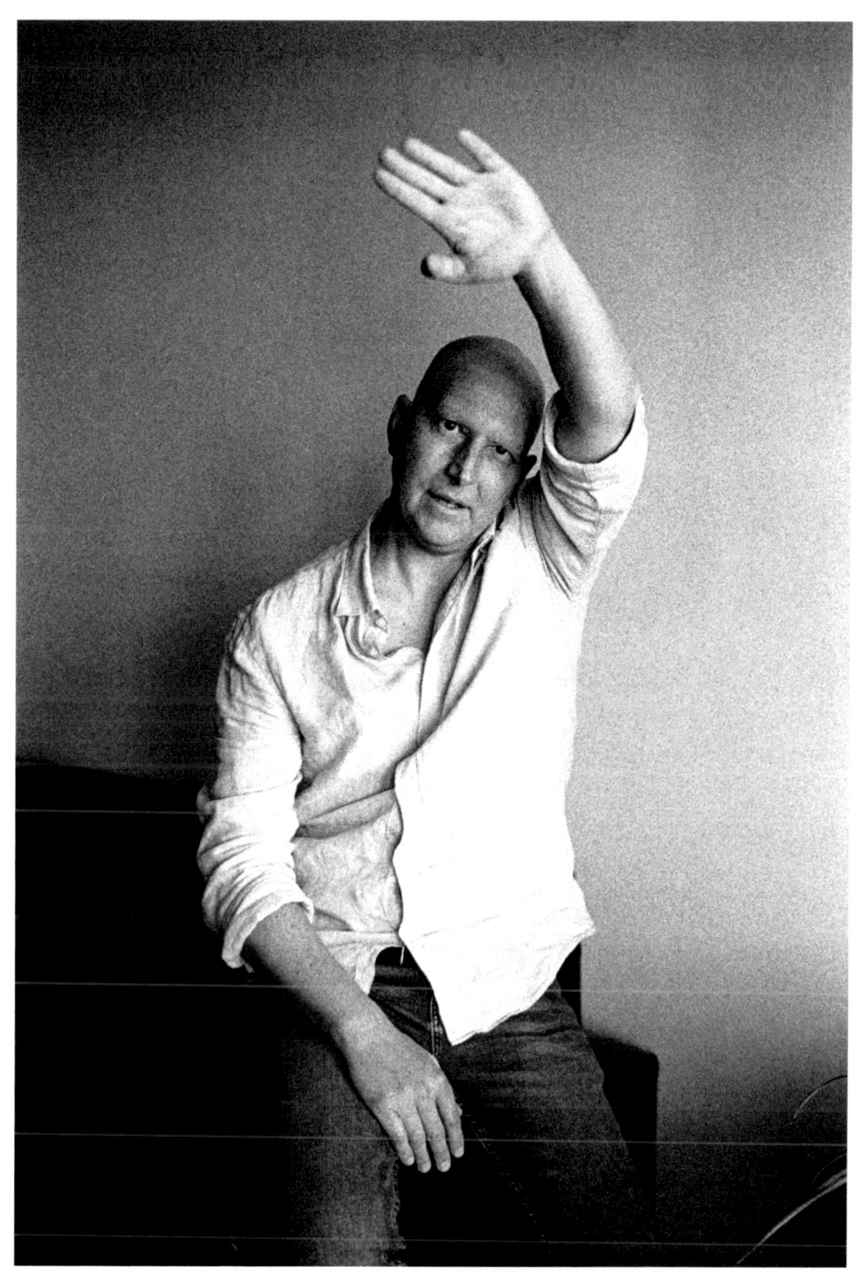

"I'm an electrical engineer. I've just turned forty. I've got a four-year-old daughter. She's the most important thing in my life at the moment.

She is still trying to get used to the fact, I've tried to explain to her that my shoulder's not well, and she says when it's better, can I hit it? I say of course, when it's better you can, all you want."

Before surgery his arm was held out for washing. The lump looked like the drawing in *The Little Prince* of a boa constrictor swallowing an elephant. And the tumour, when they'd cut it out, was a gnarled, knobbly thing, like something the dog might have dug up. It was left lying on the table, next to the red threads that tie muslin swabs in bundles of five, placed there carefully to be counted at the end.

All the tumours I photographed were different.

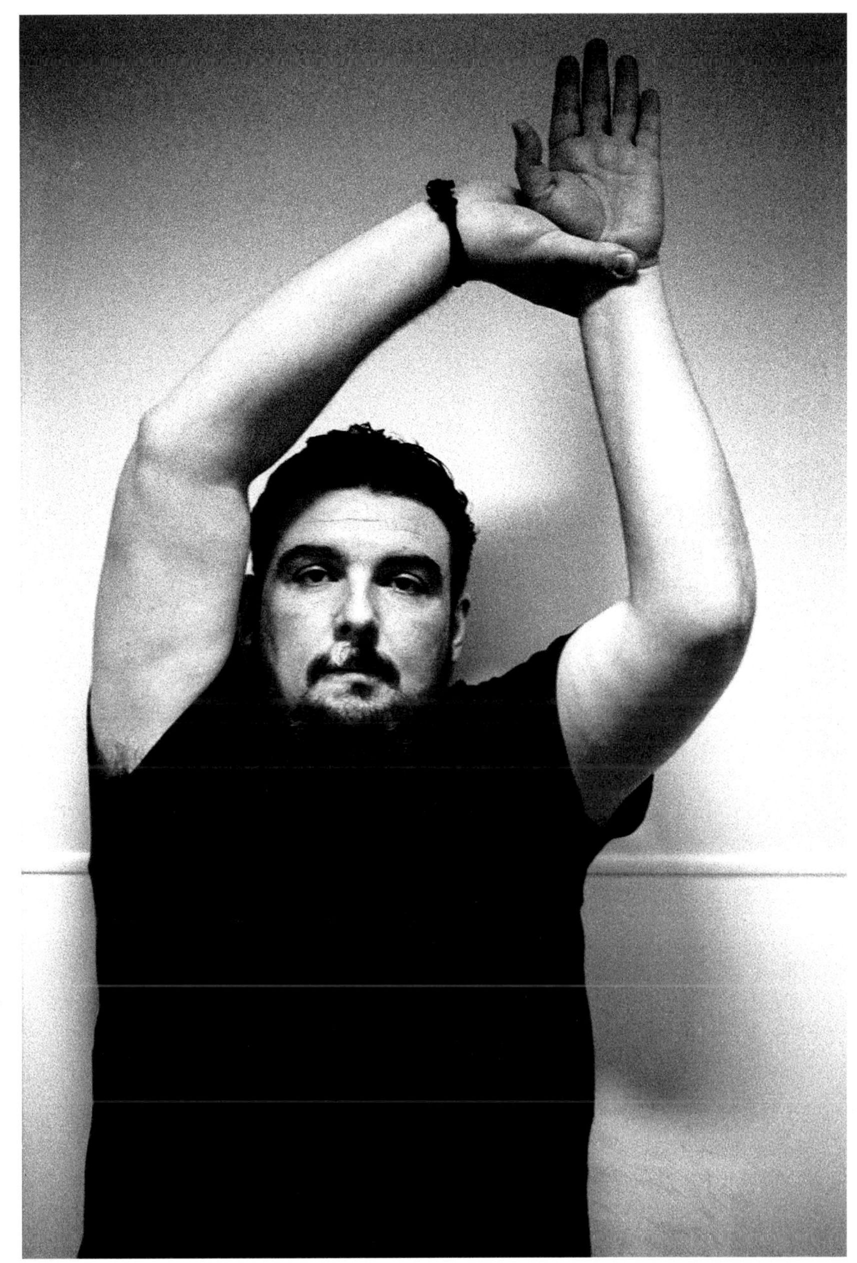

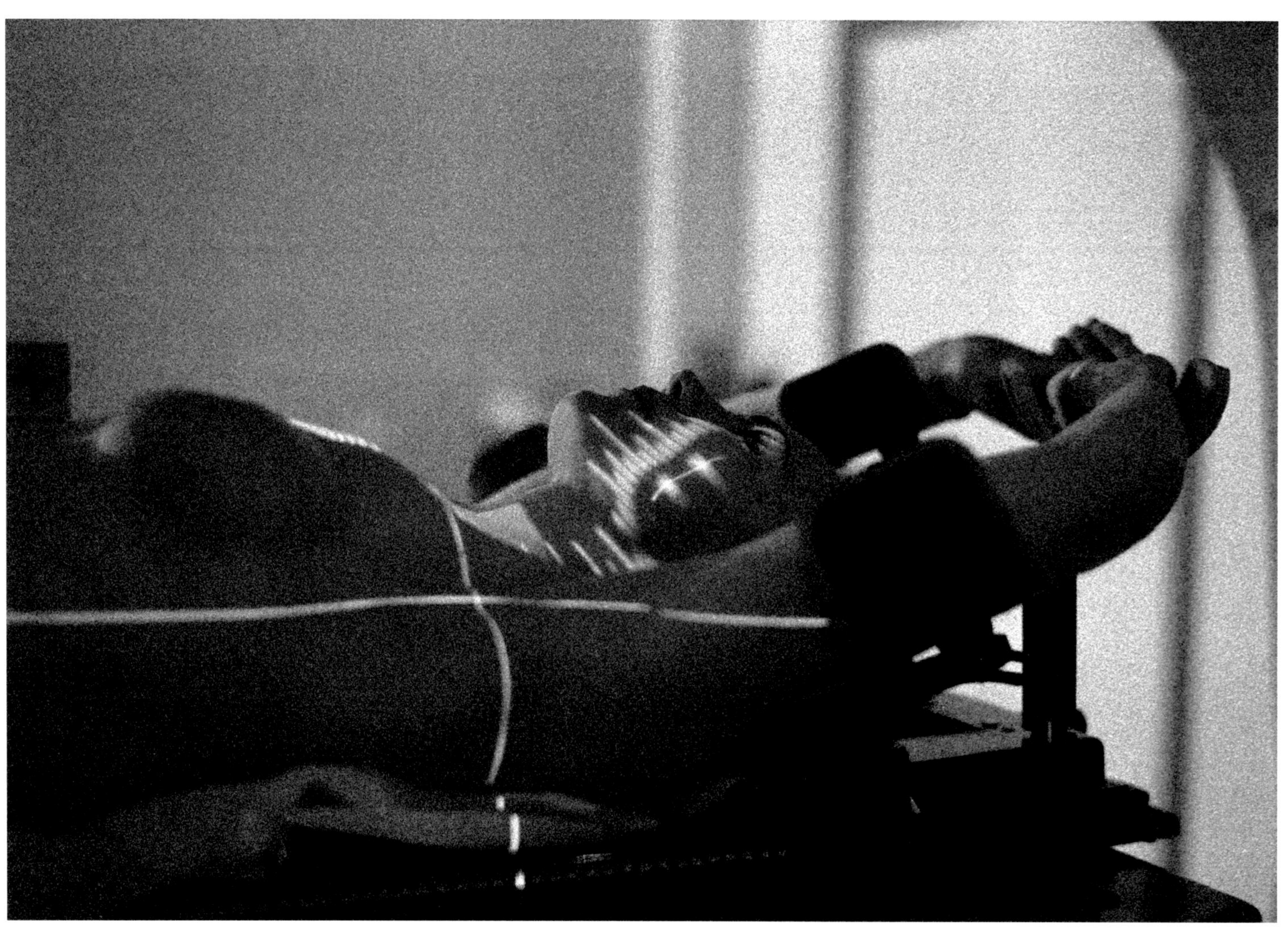

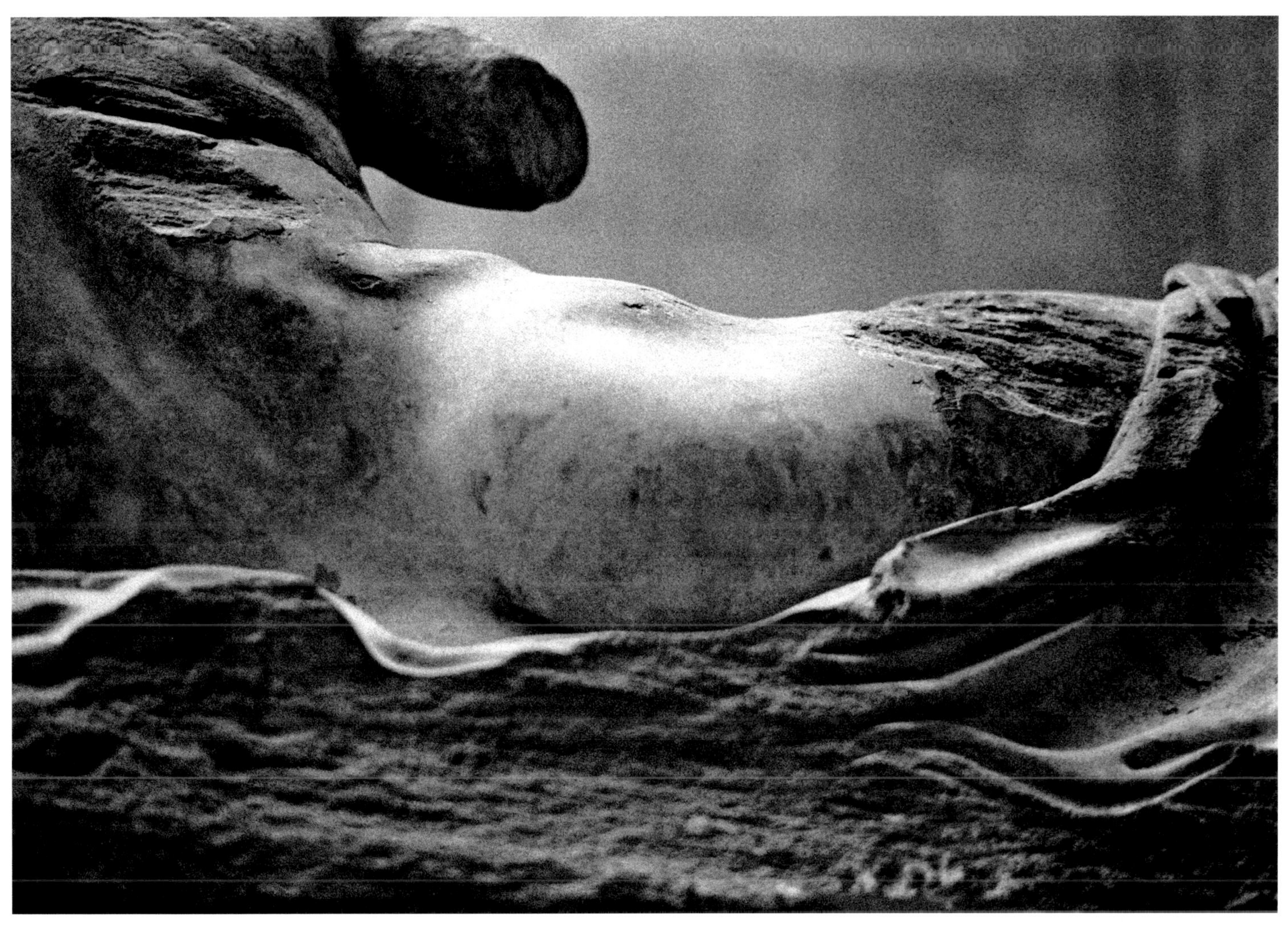

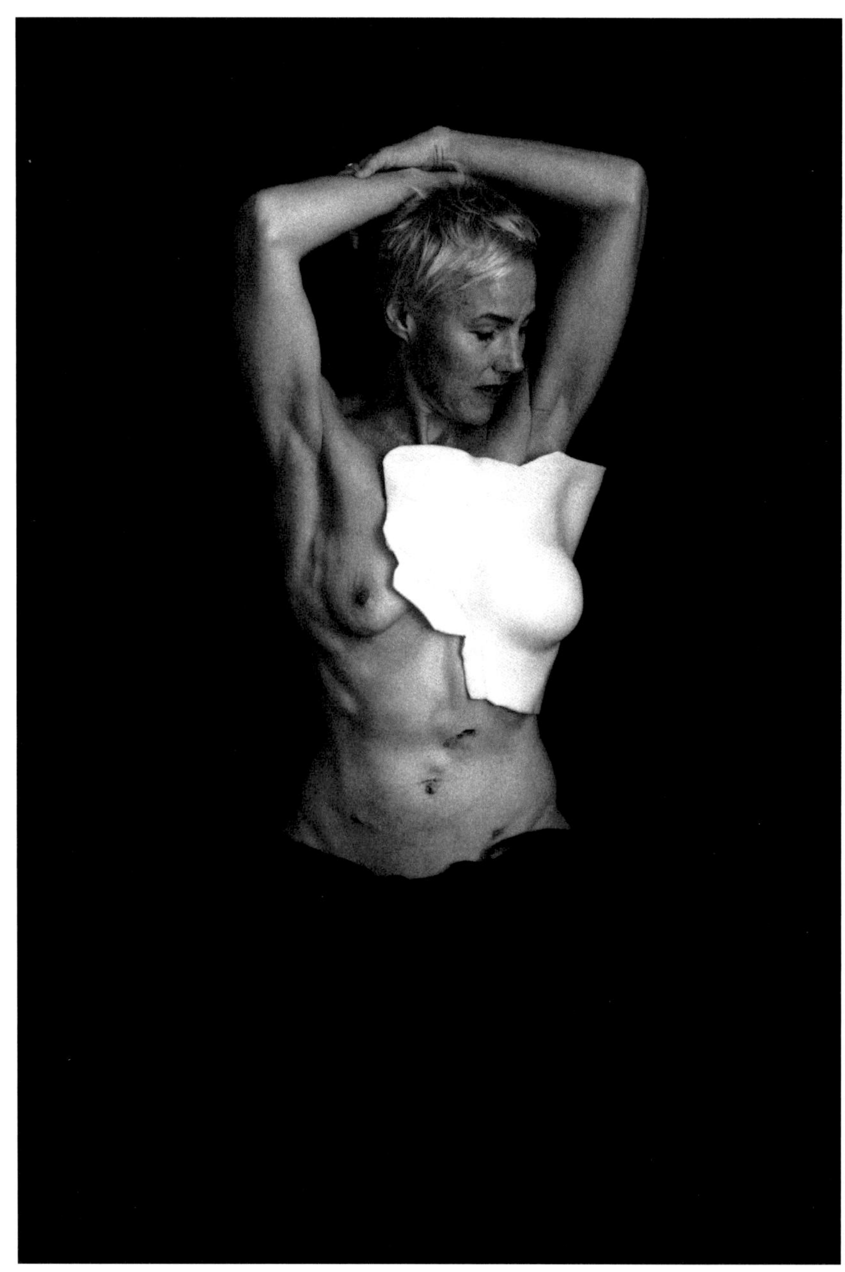

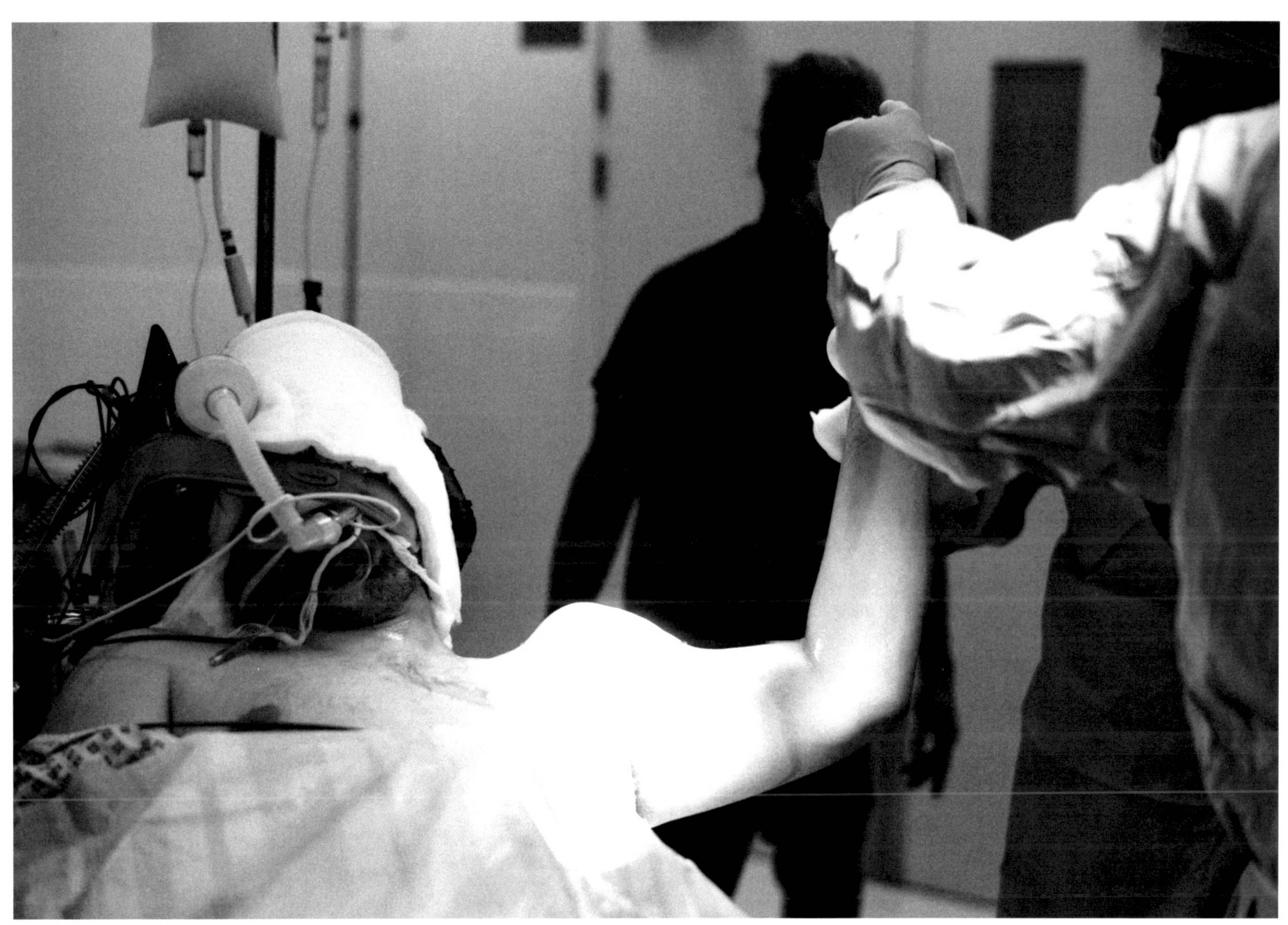

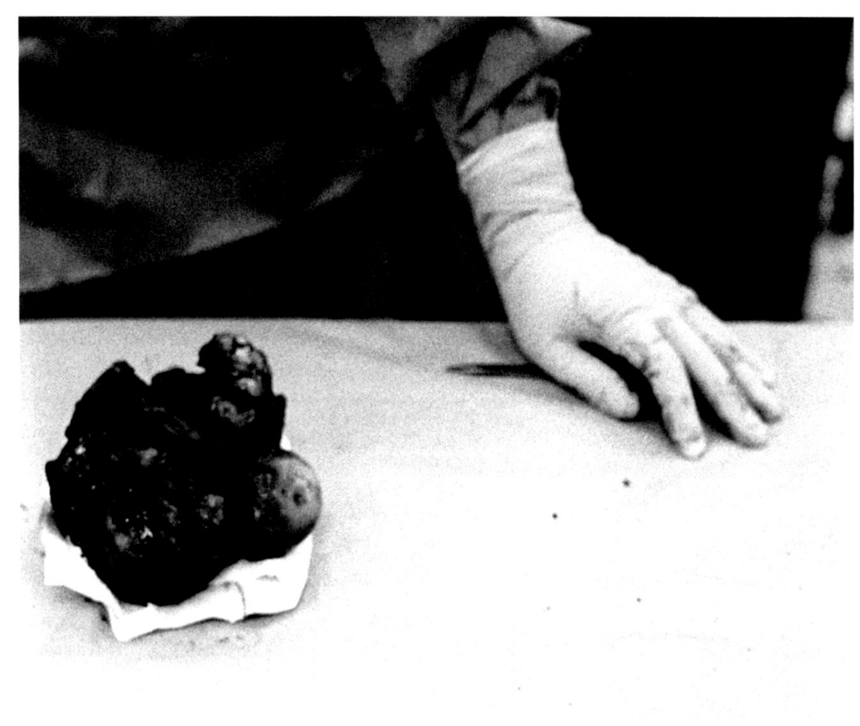

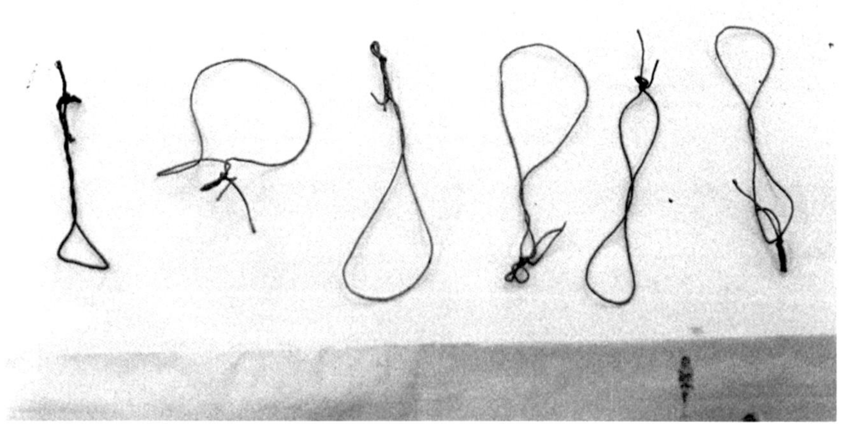

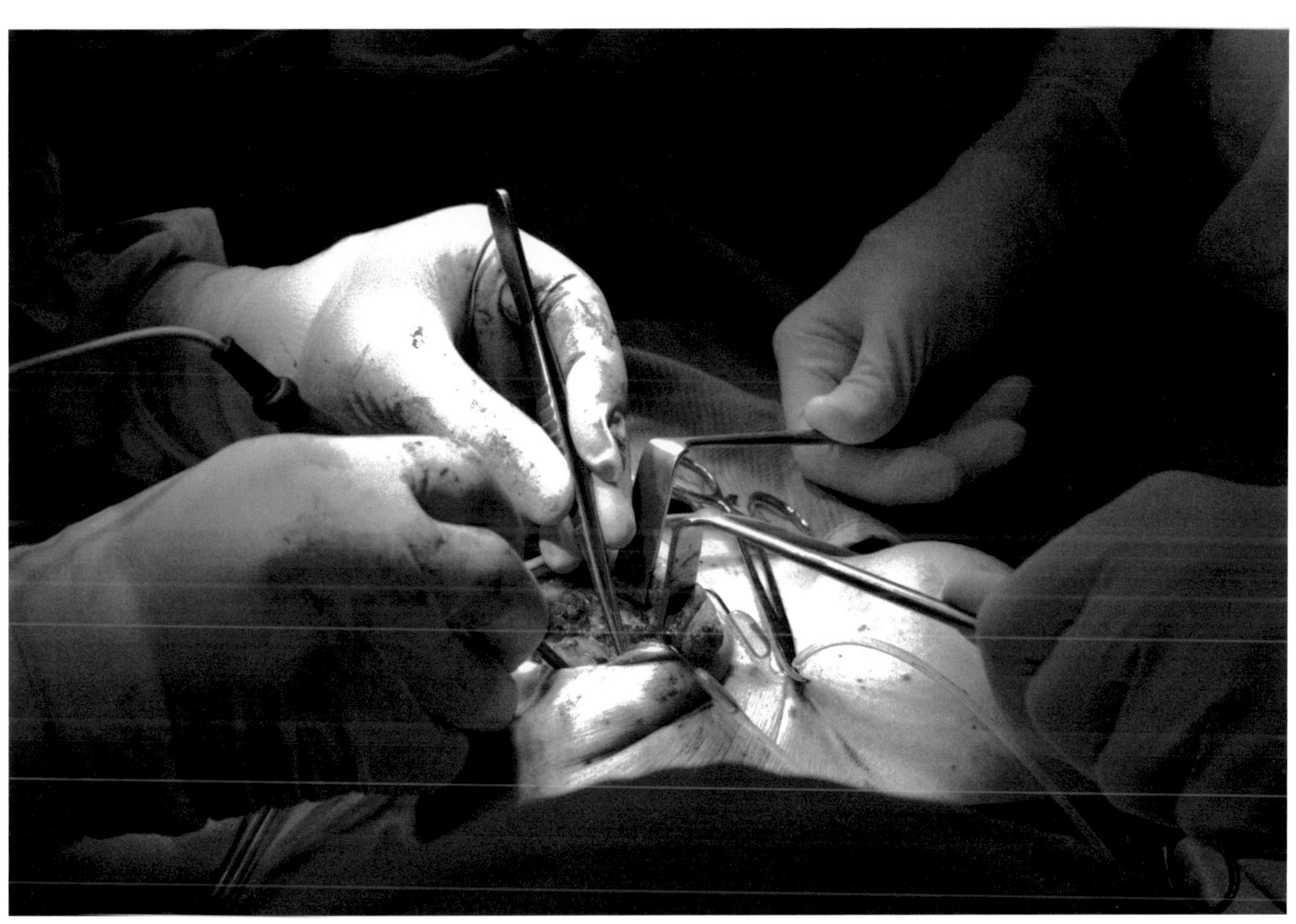

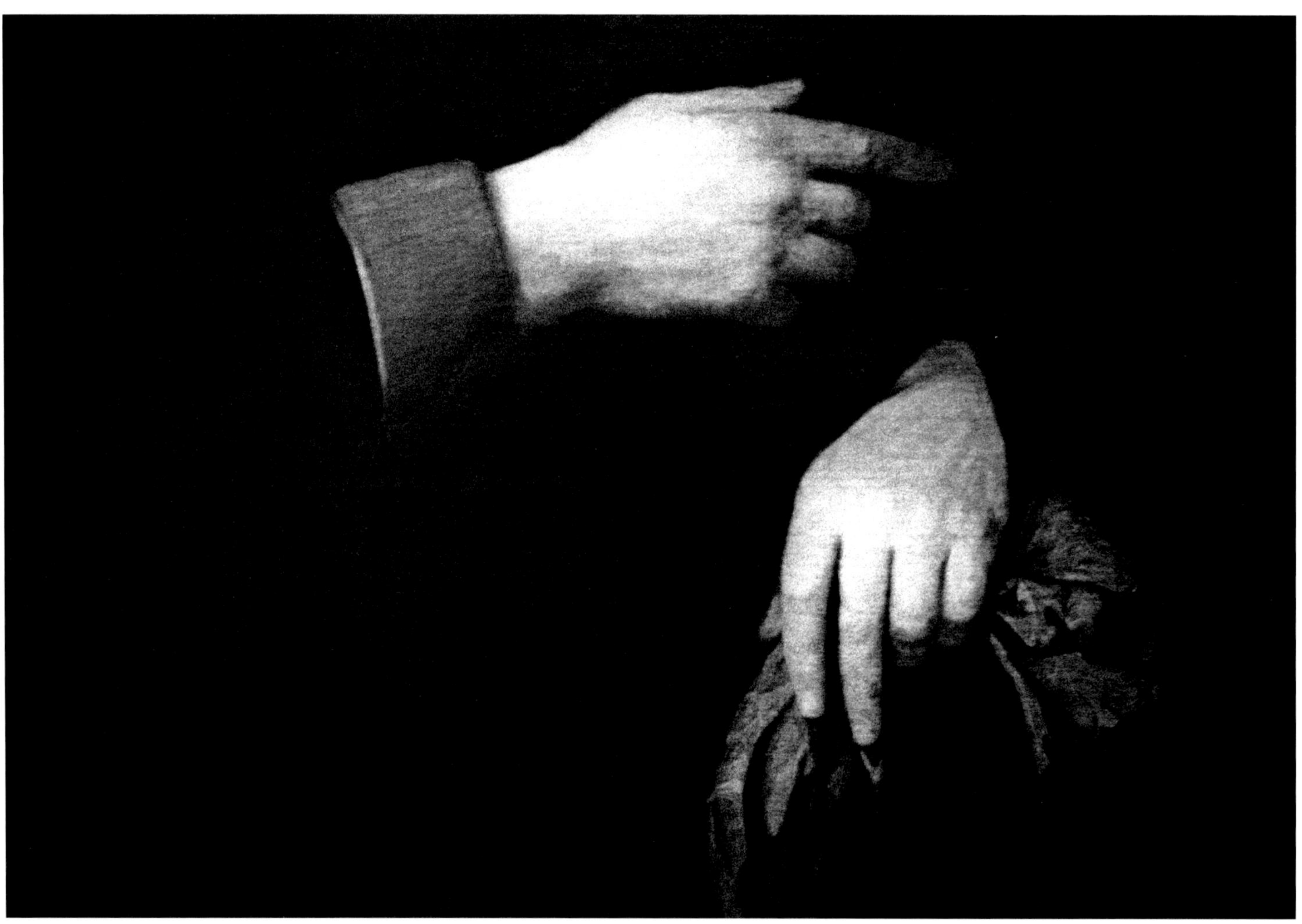

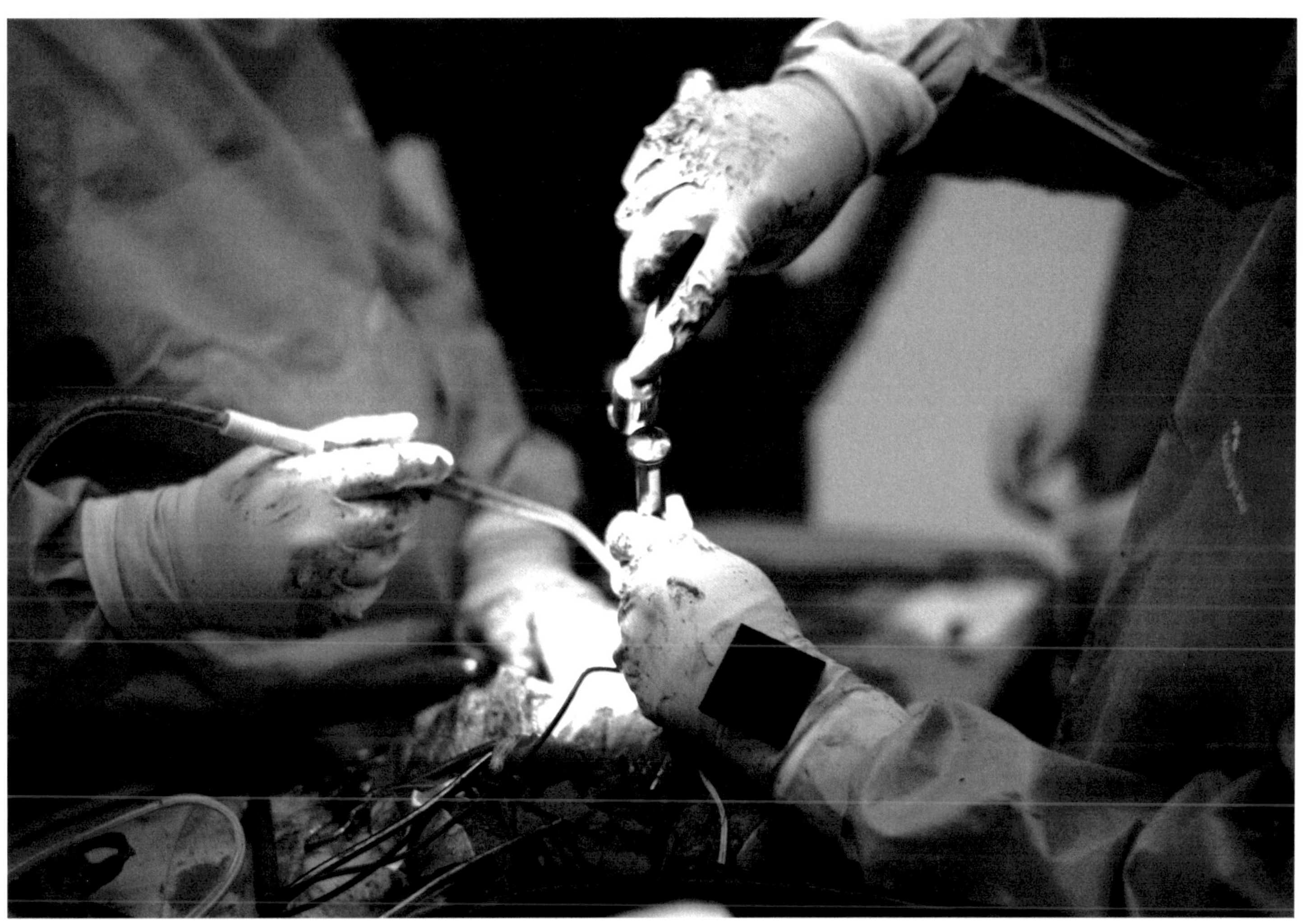

"So after I gave birth to Theo, I was with my mum and we were planning to go out for lunch. We were trying to fit the Isofit base into the car for the car seat and my mum couldn't do it and said 'I know you've not long given birth, but can you try and do it?' So I went out and I remember pushing it, and it was hot, it was a lovely summer day. I was pushing and pushing and it wouldn't go in.

I pushed to the point where I remember hearing this crunch in my left arm. And I remember thinking 'Oh my god, my arm, I've really hurt it'.

The surgeon explained it was osteo-sarcoma, and what that was, and told me the plan was for me to go straight in as soon as possible because they found the fracture in my arm. The bone had snapped because of the pressure from the tumour growing on it."

Surgery is planned, controlled and sanctioned violence, to prevent a greater harm.

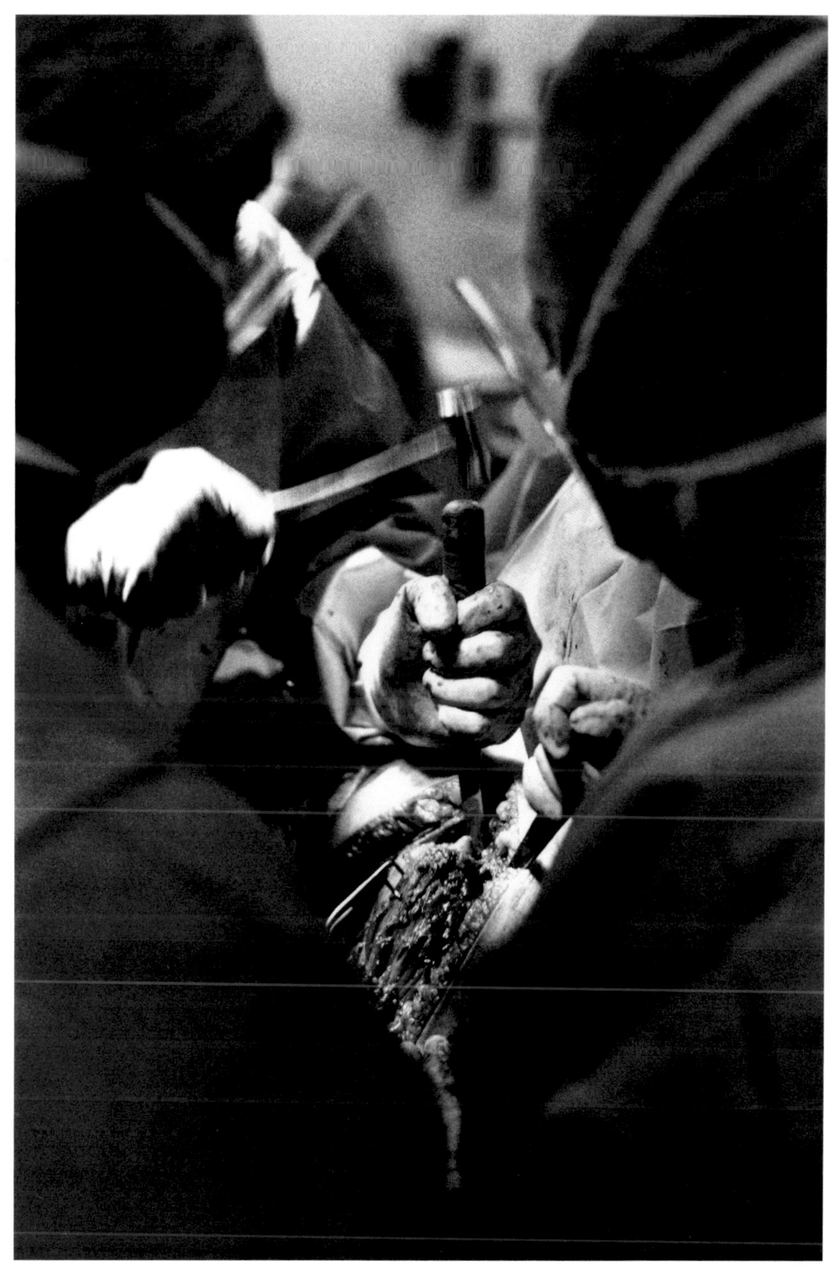

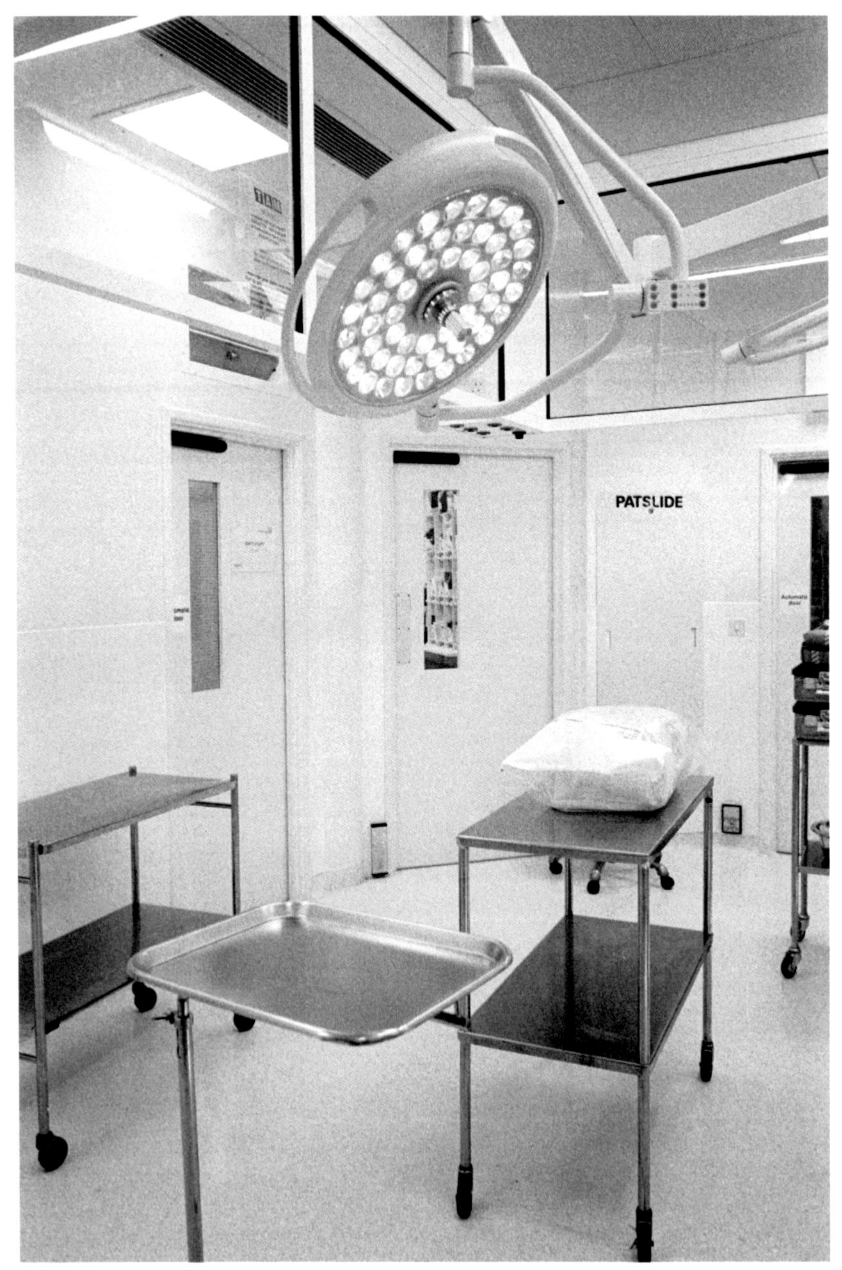
PATSLIDE

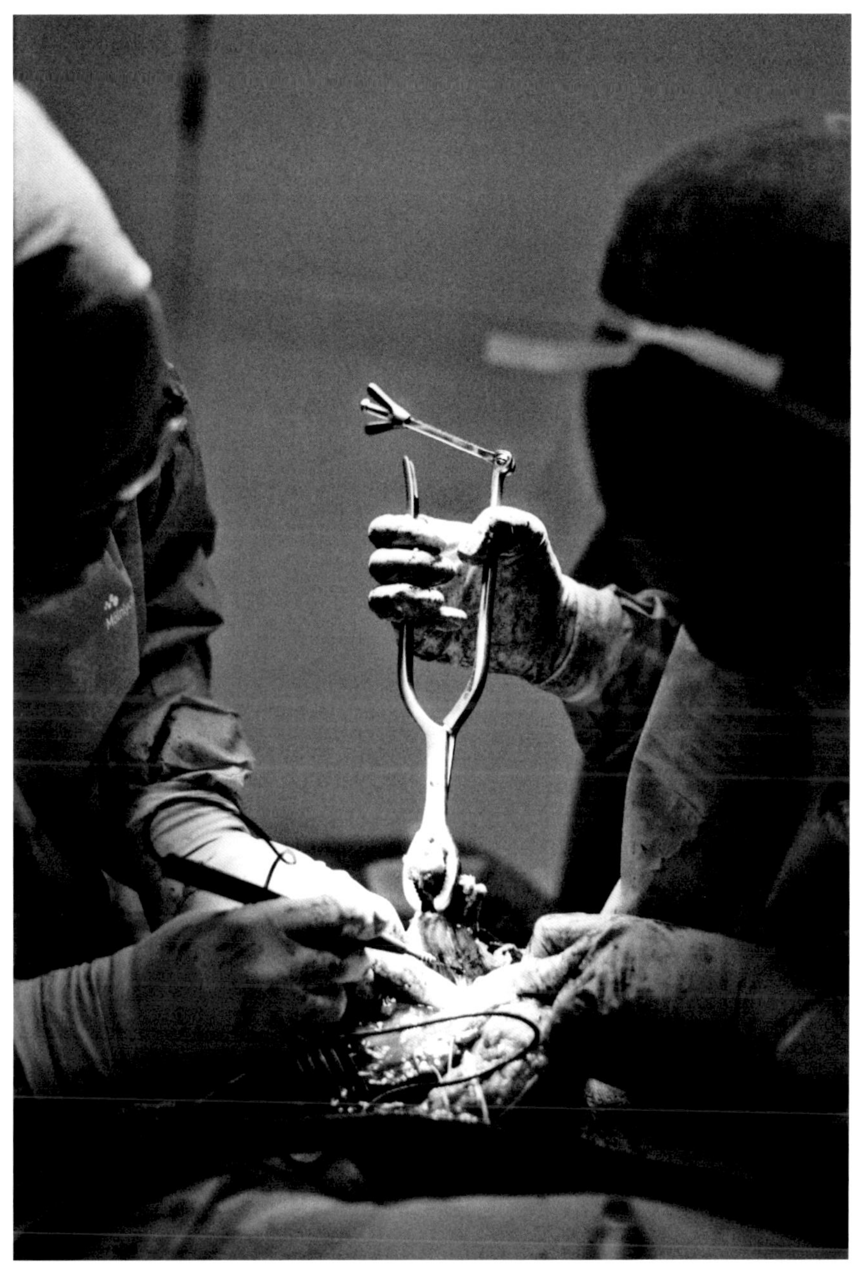

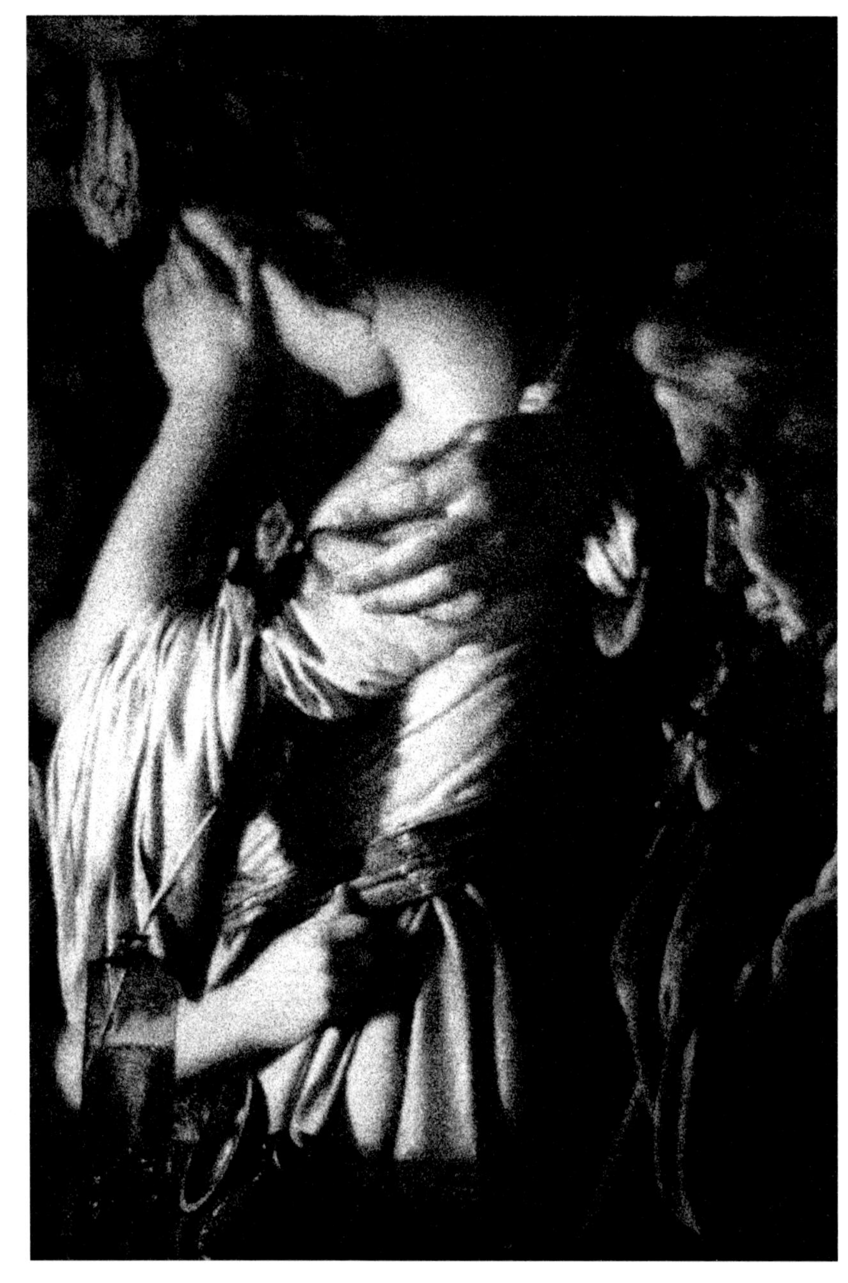

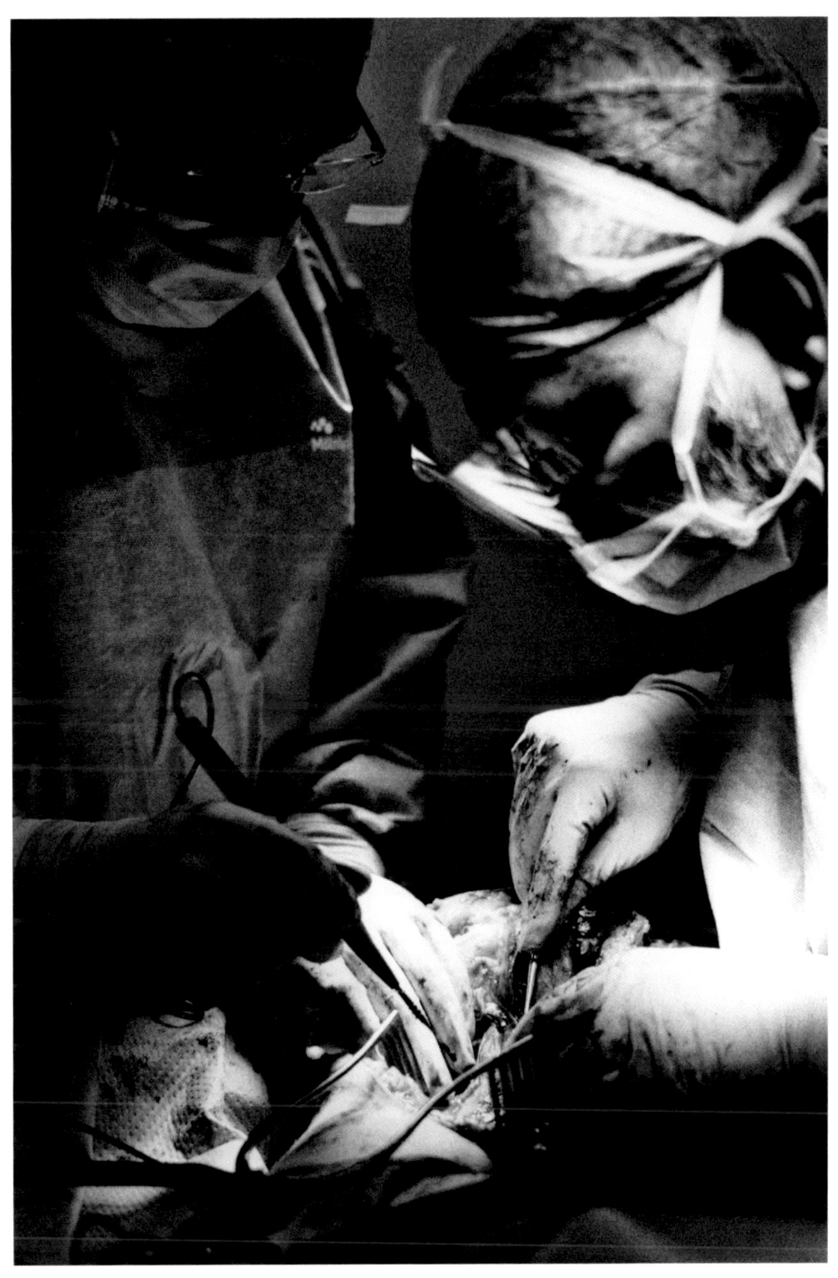

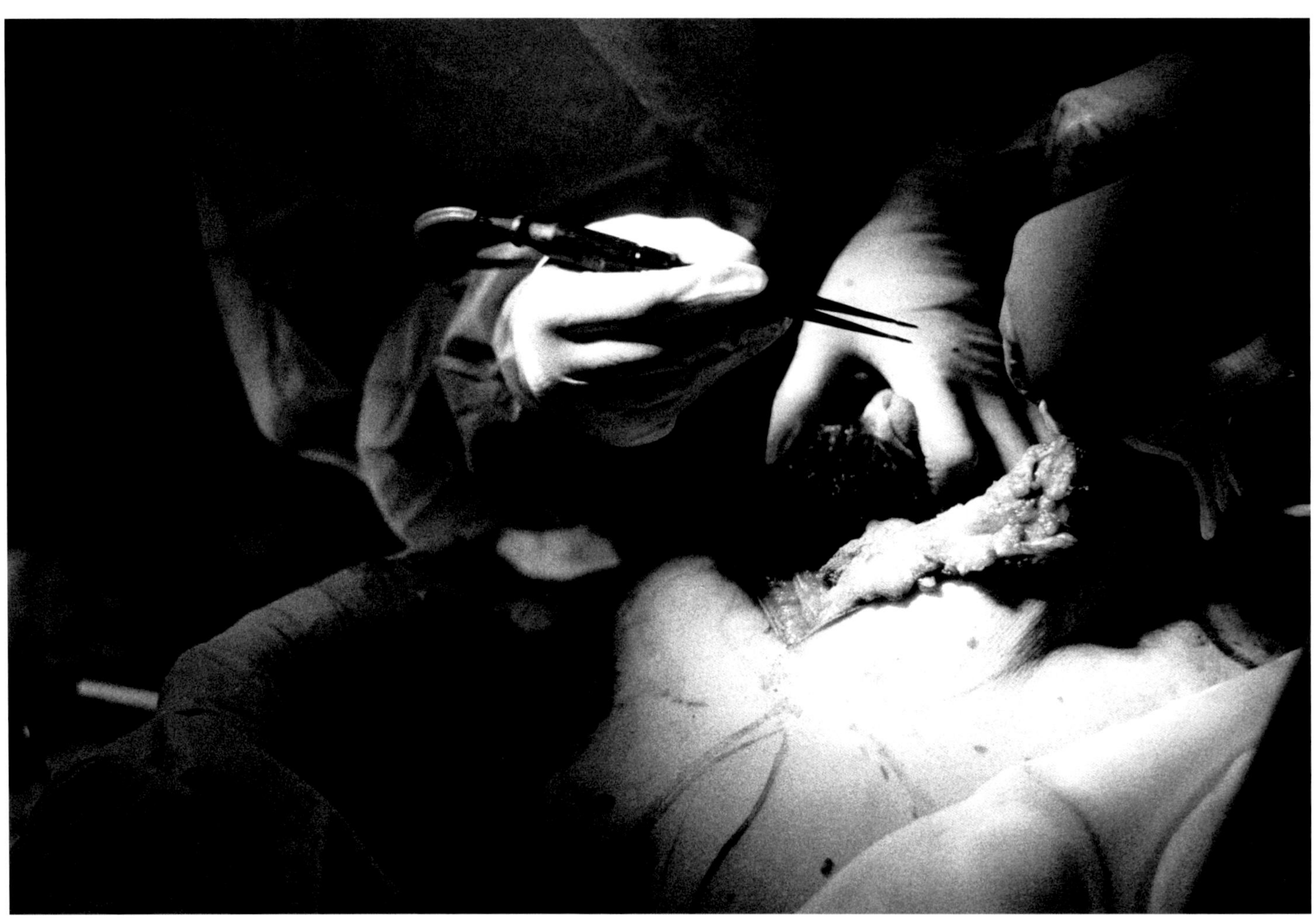

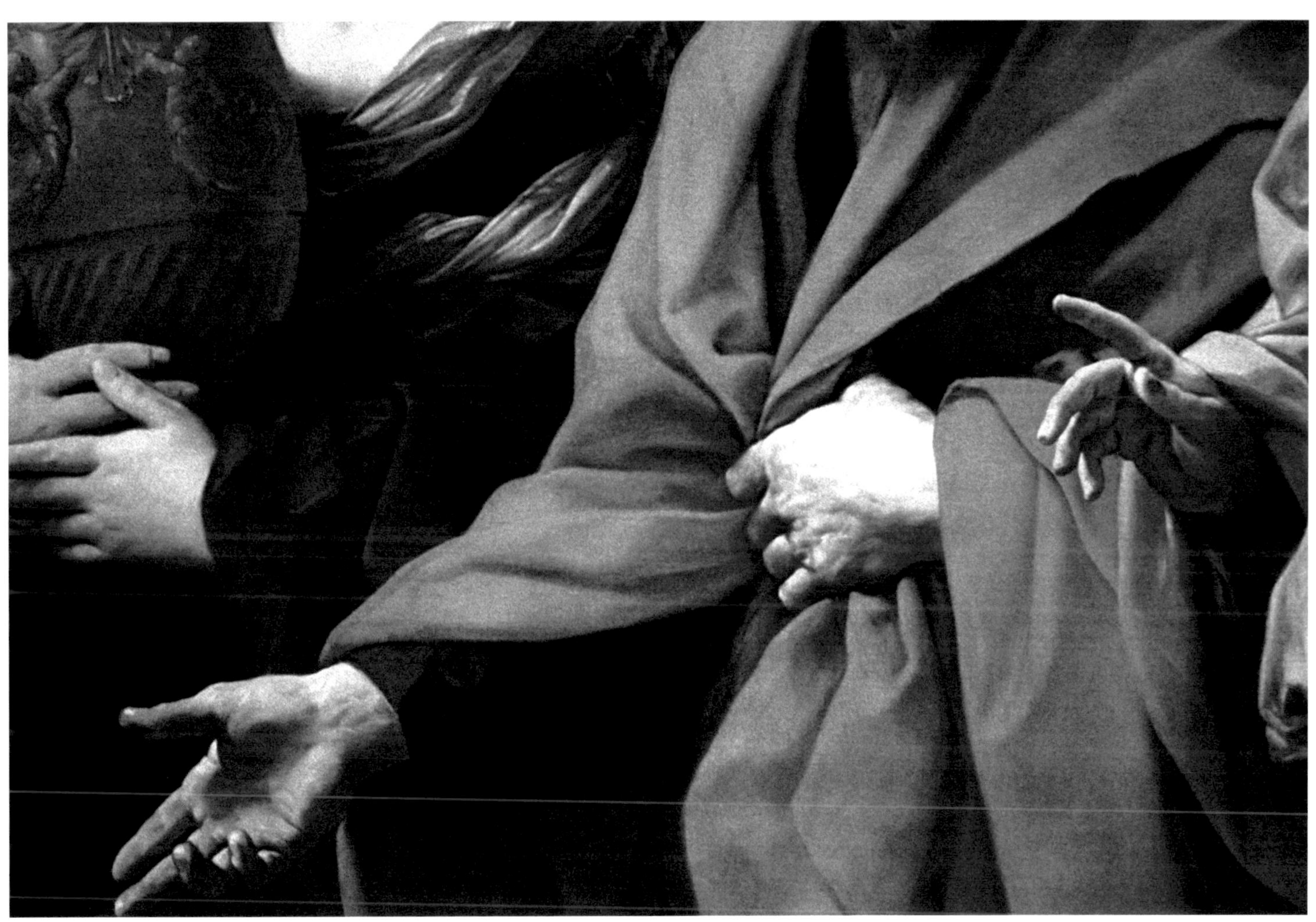

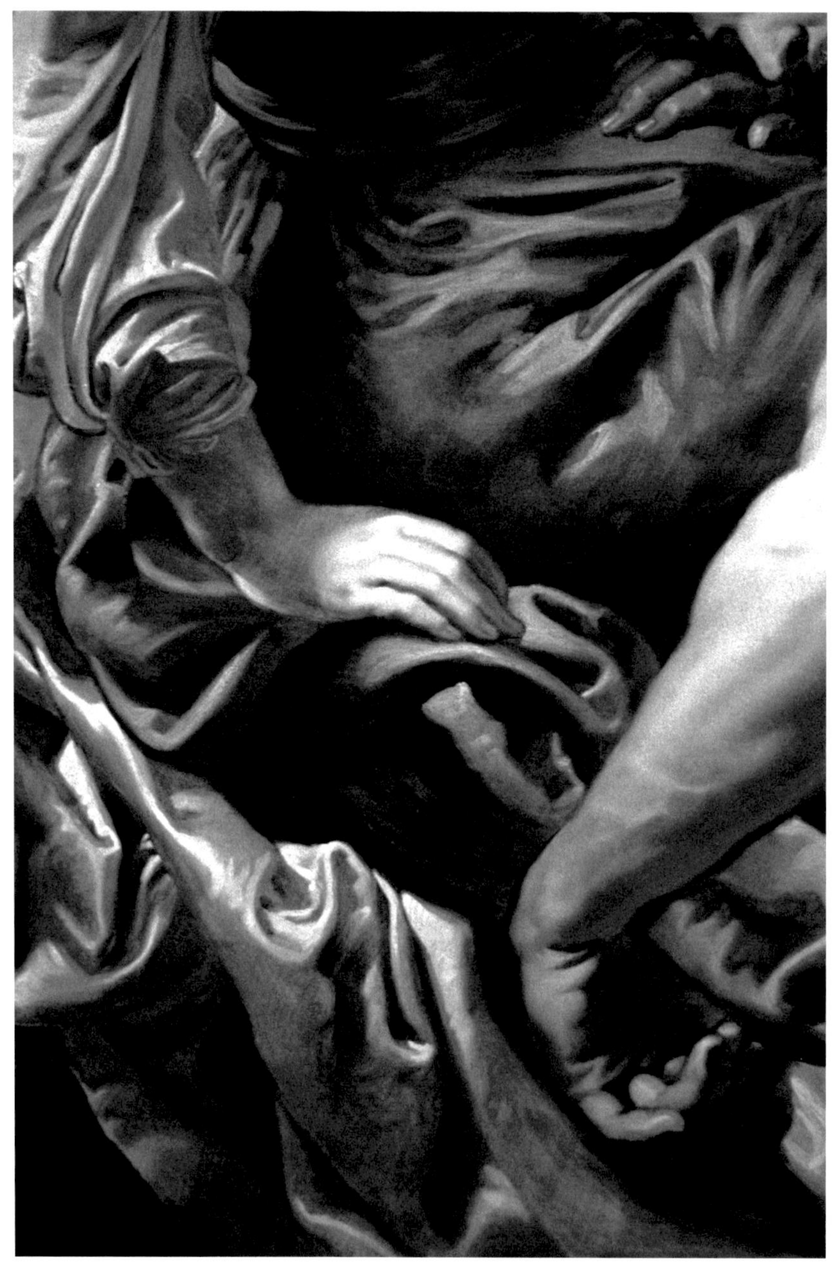

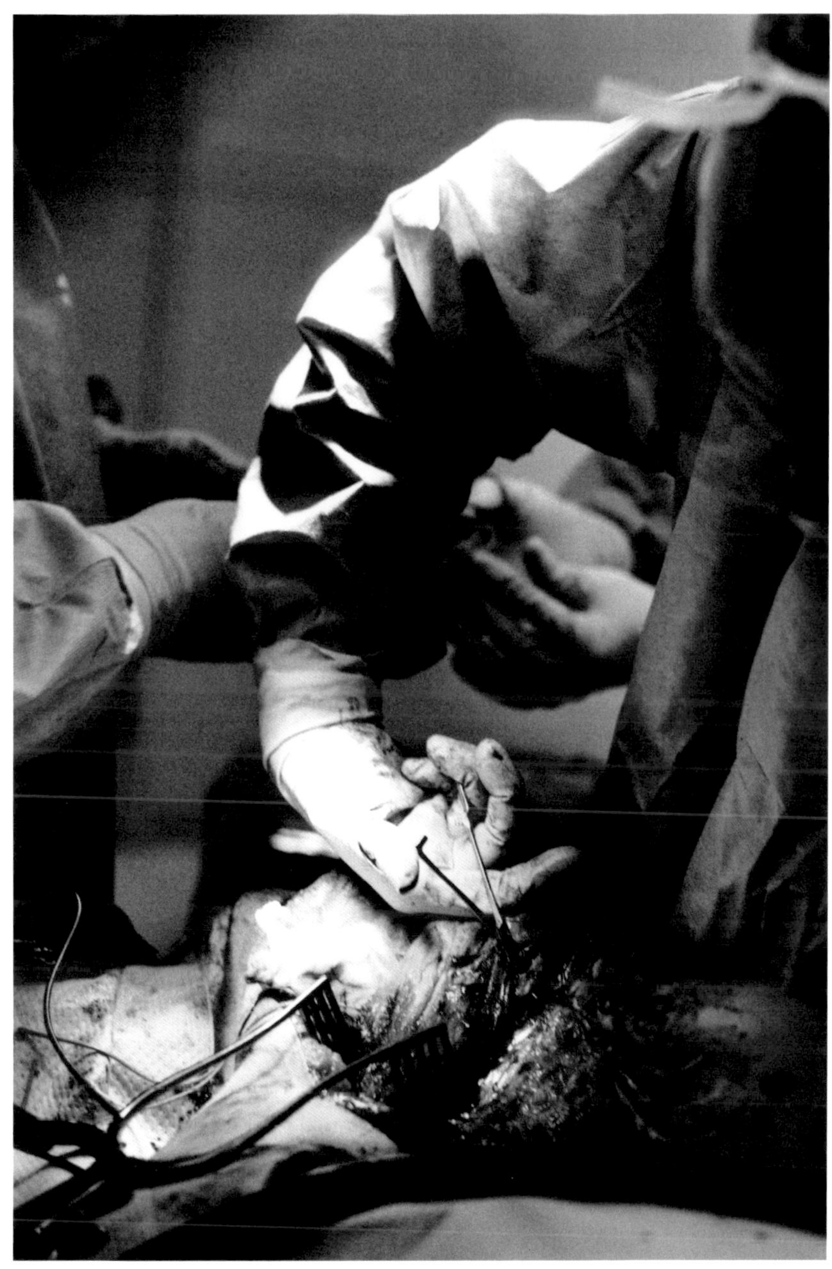

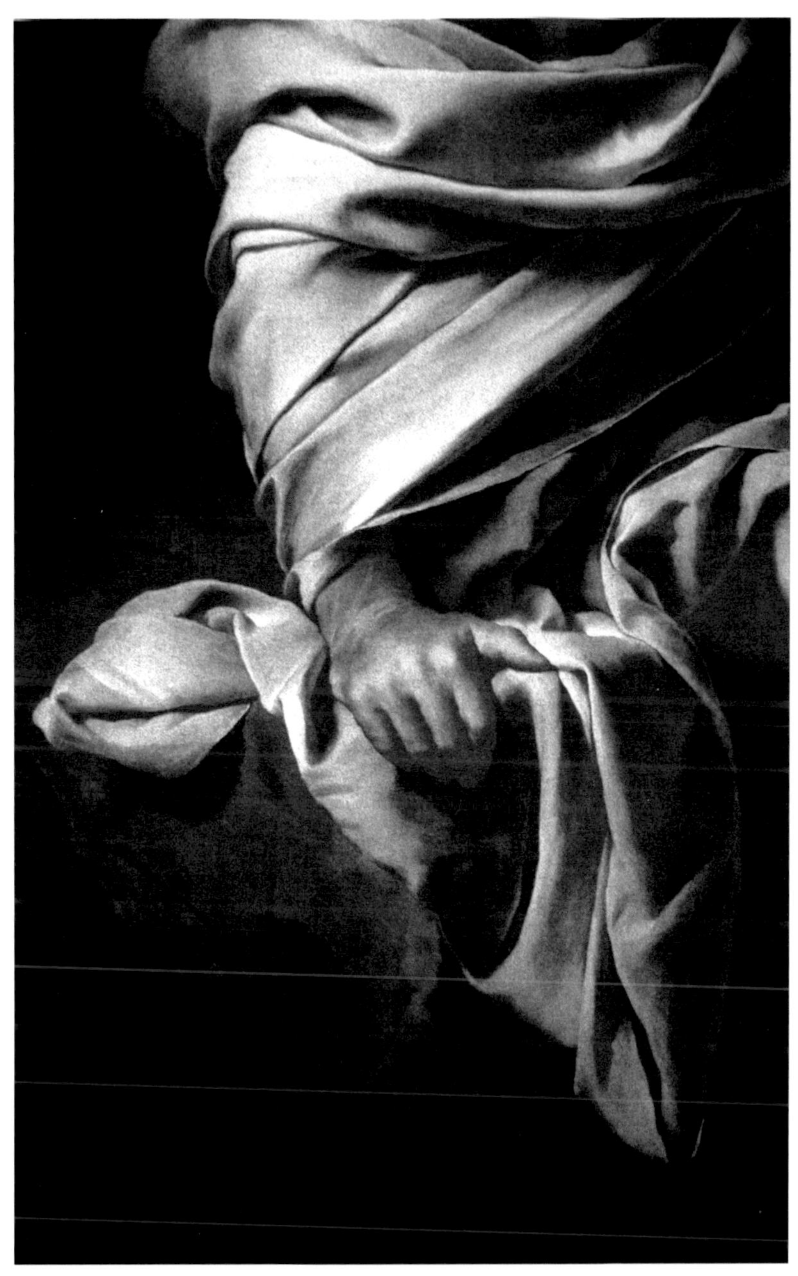

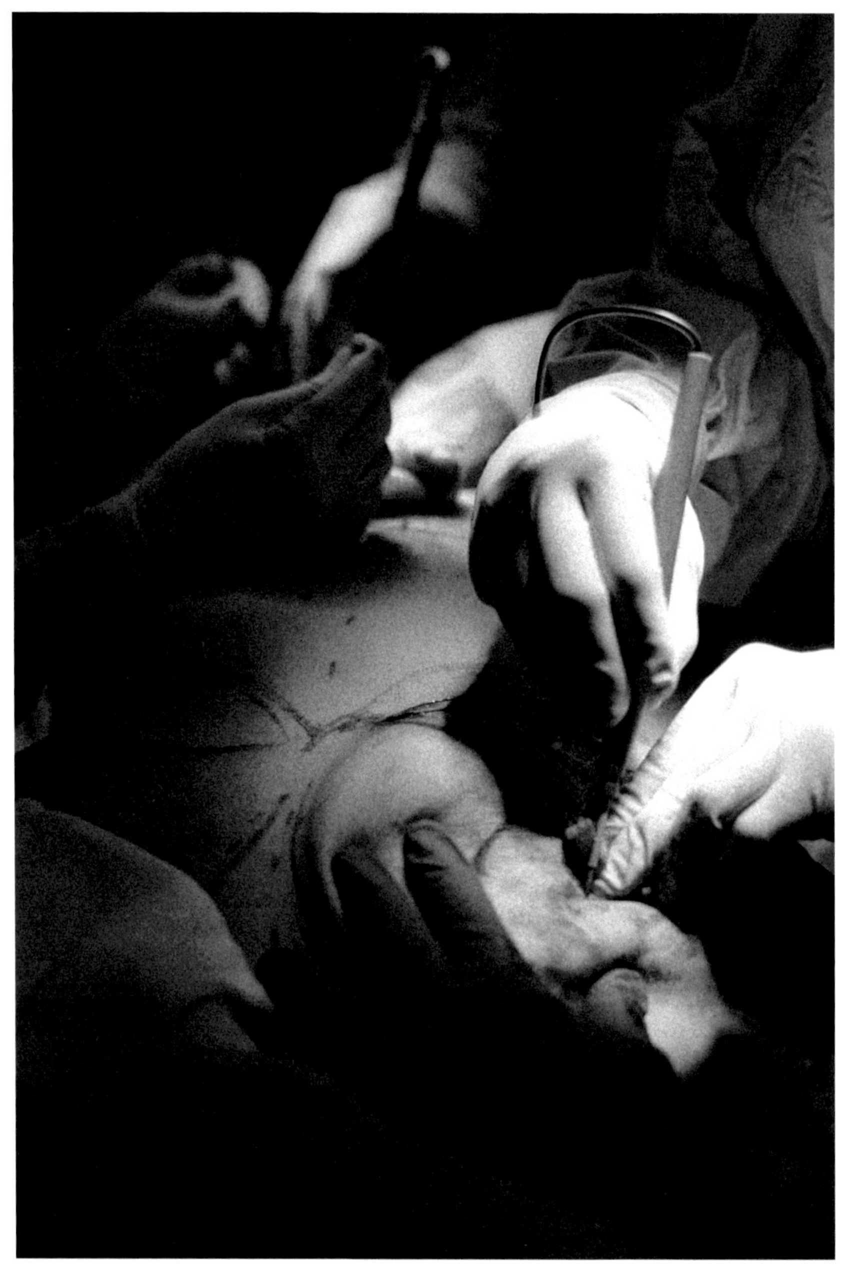

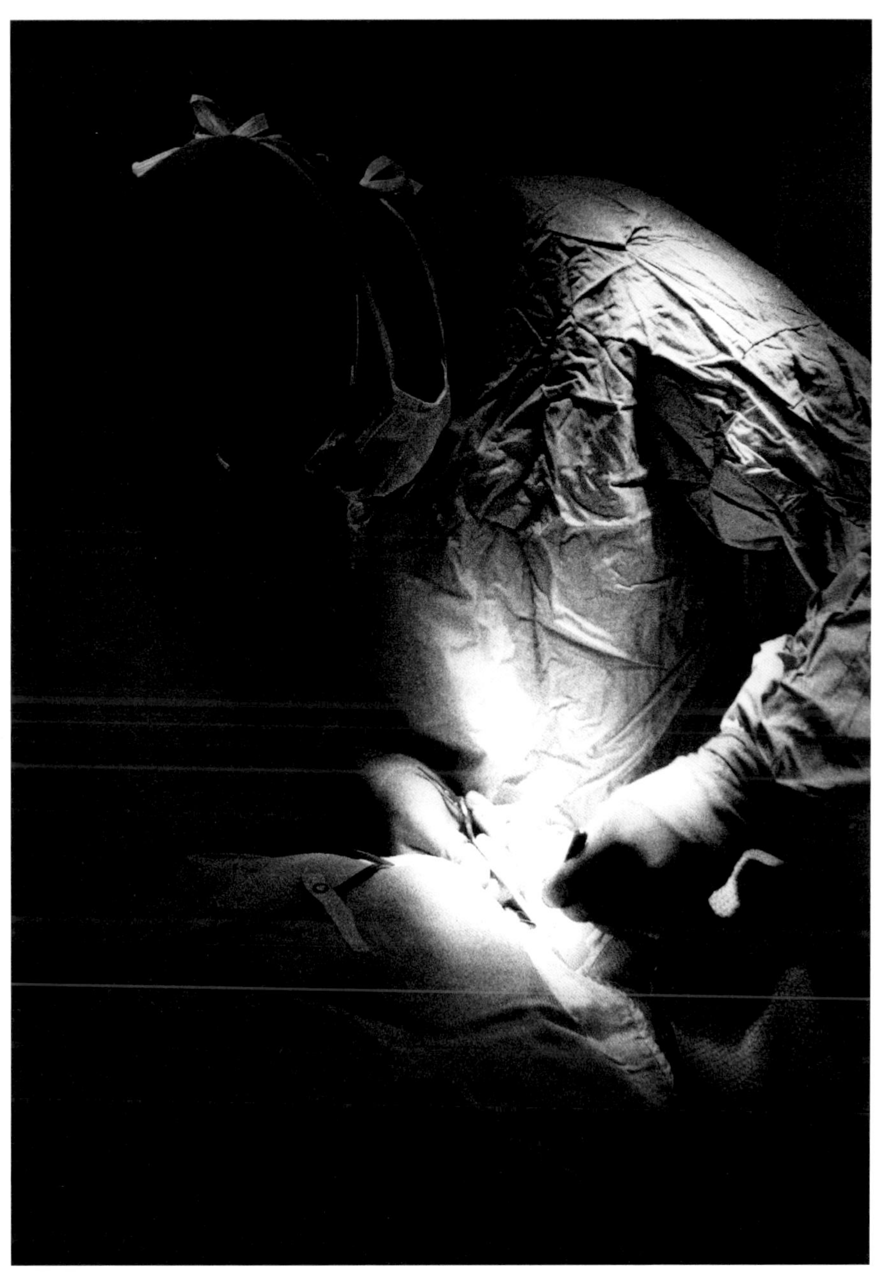

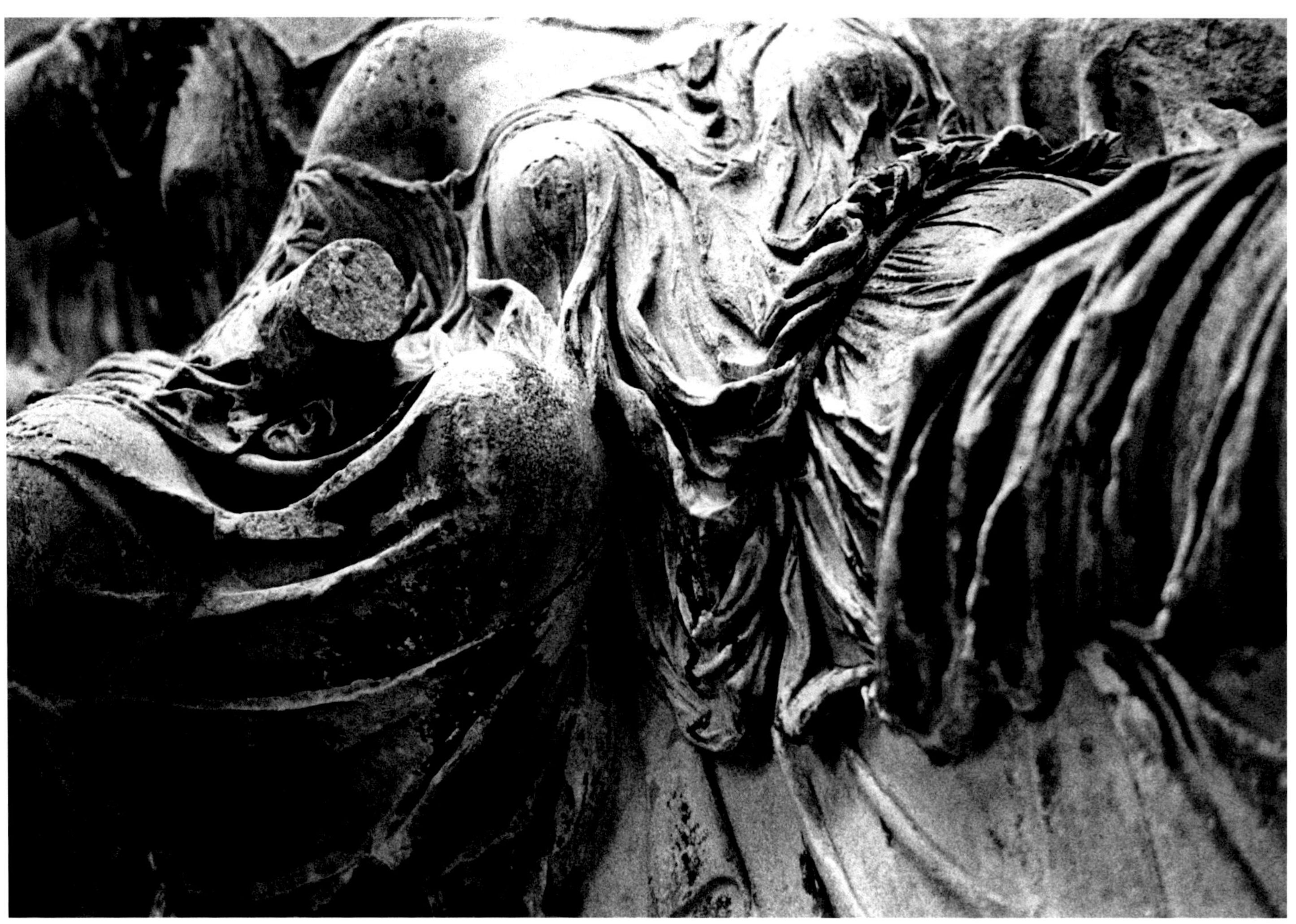

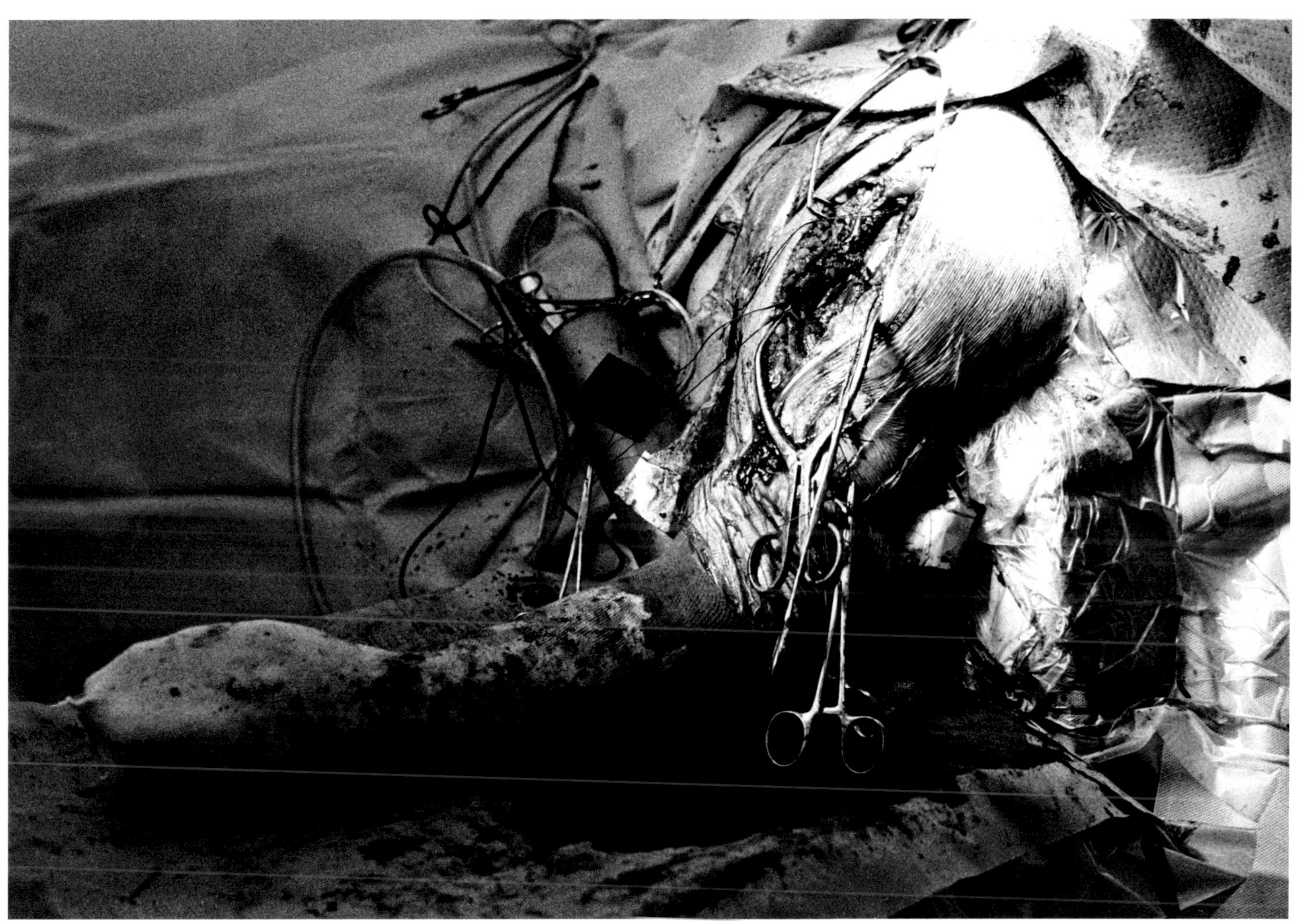

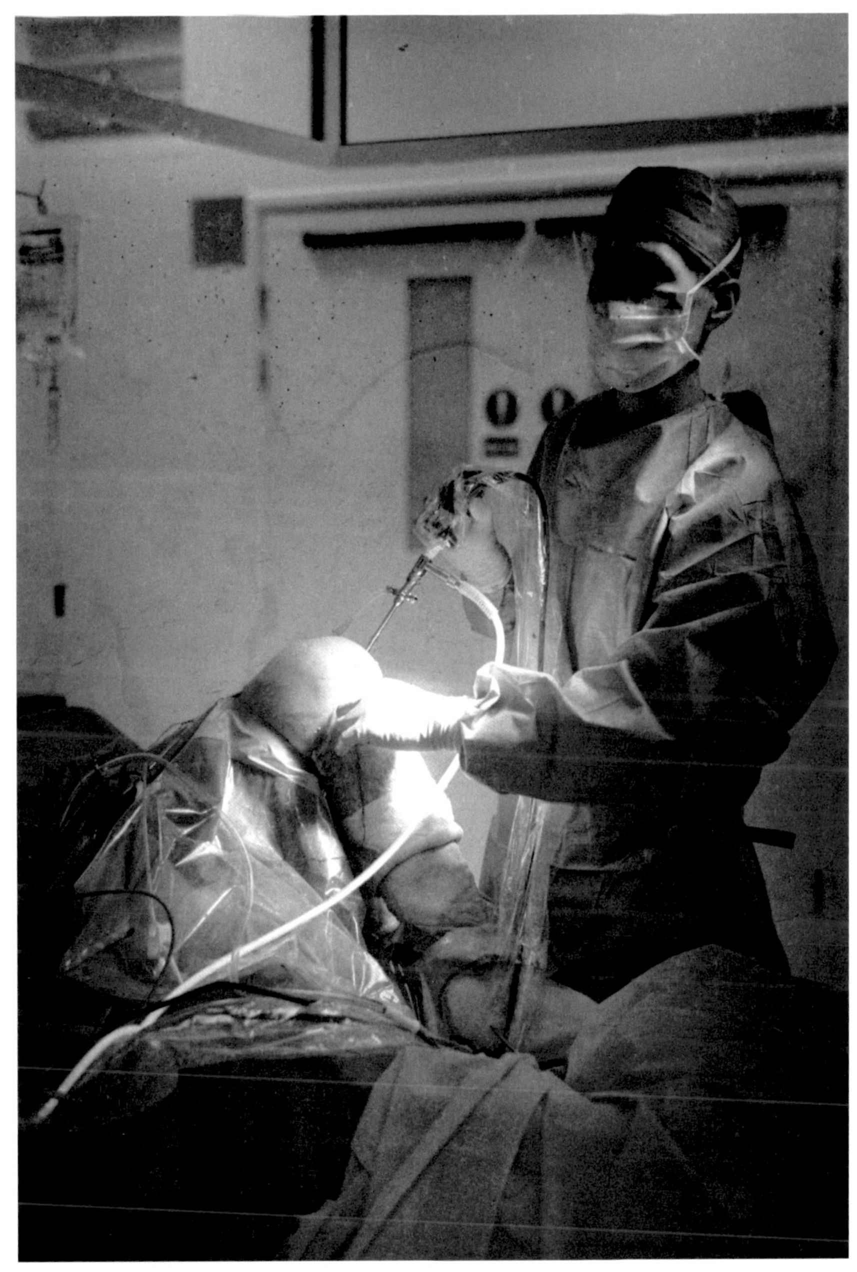

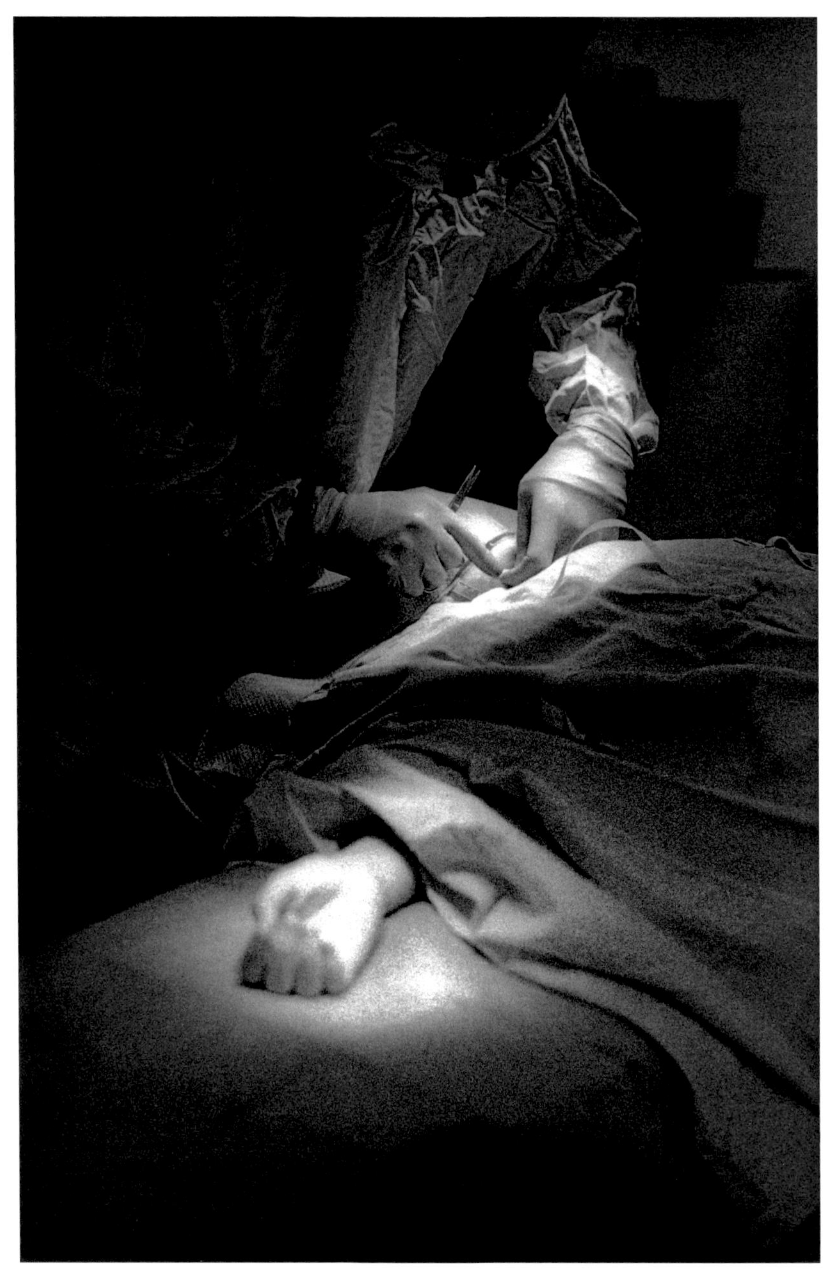

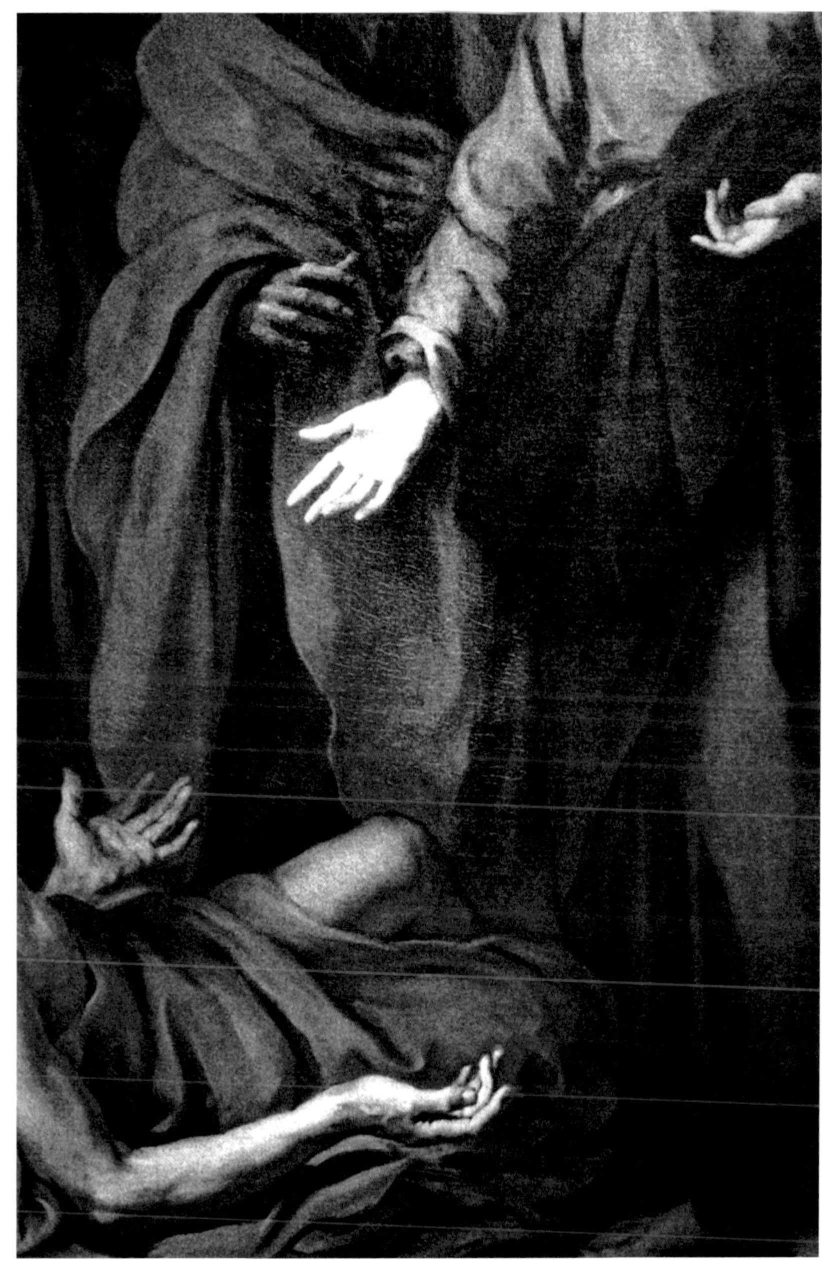

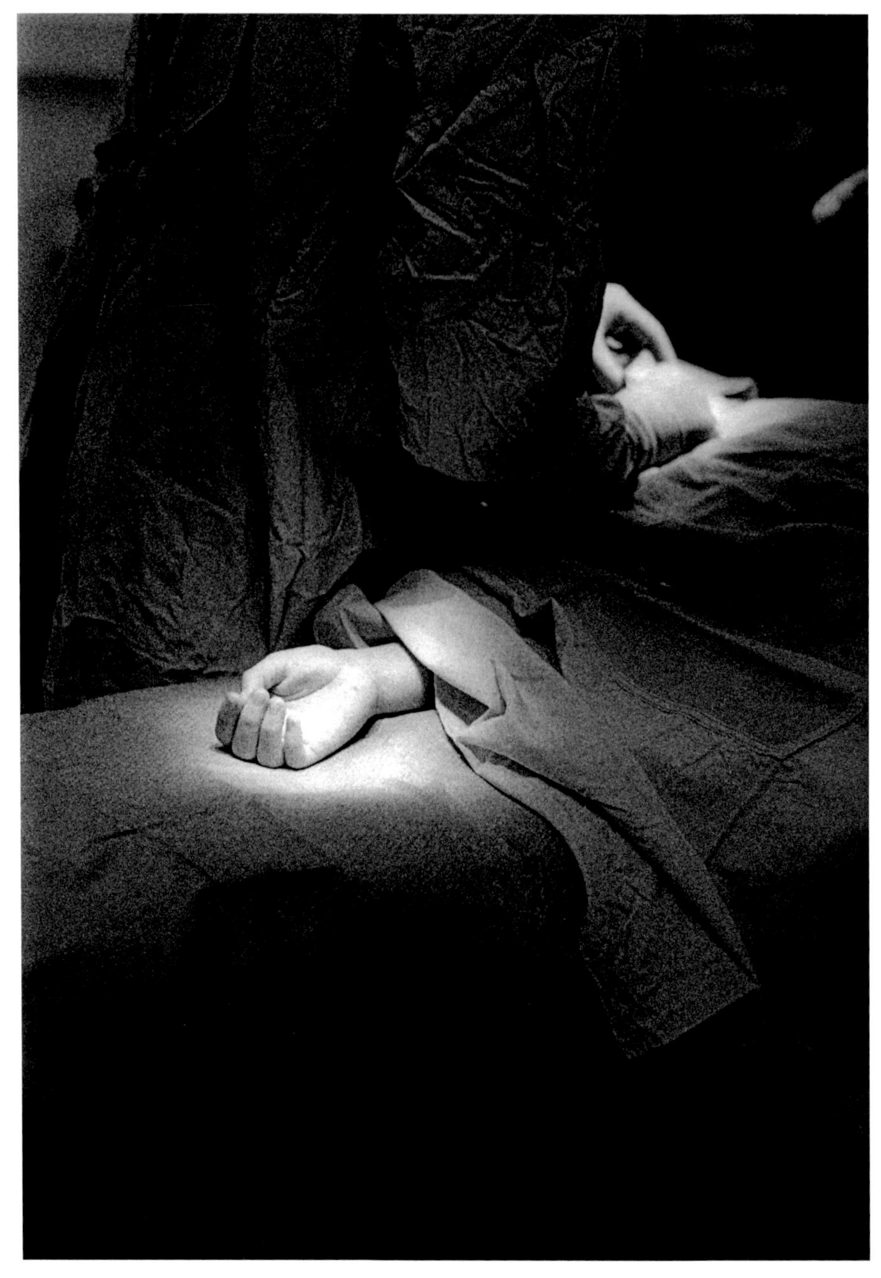

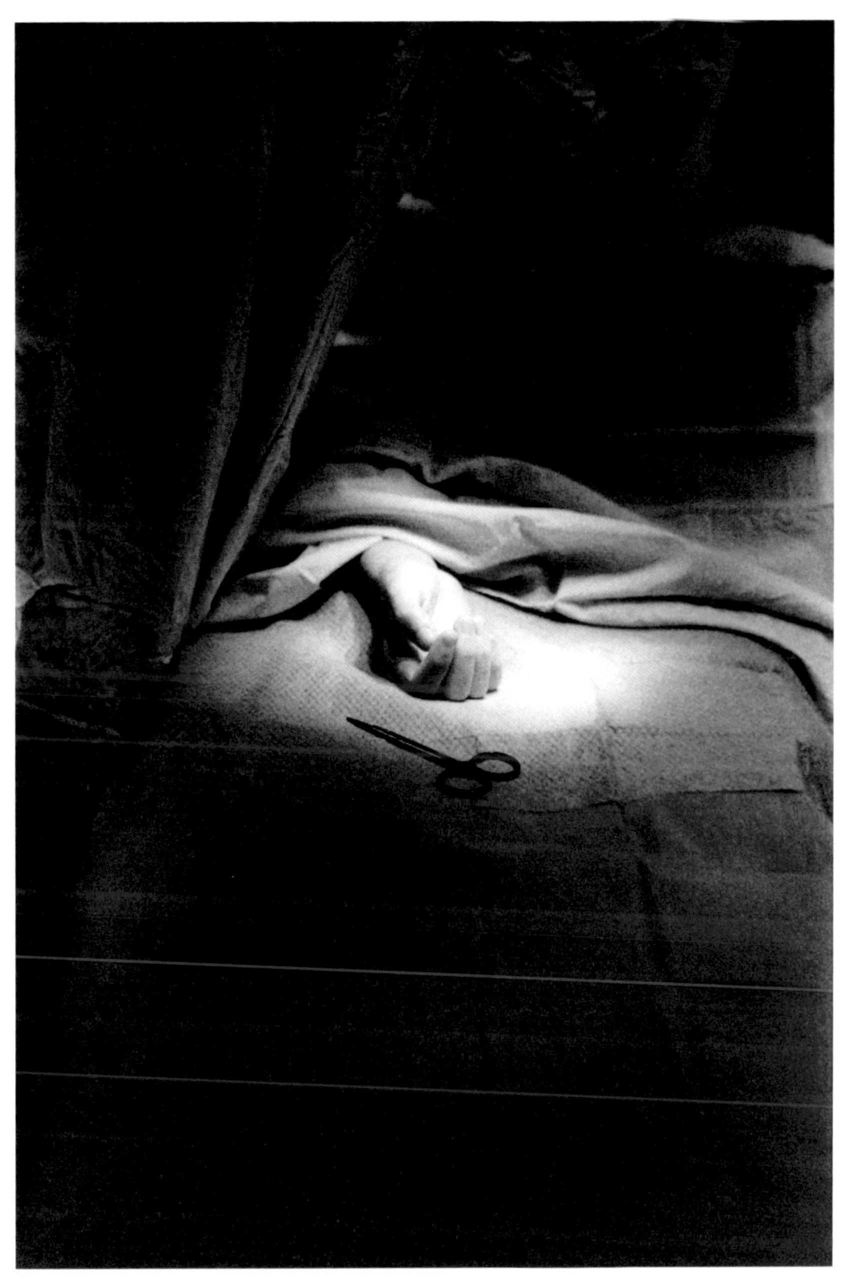

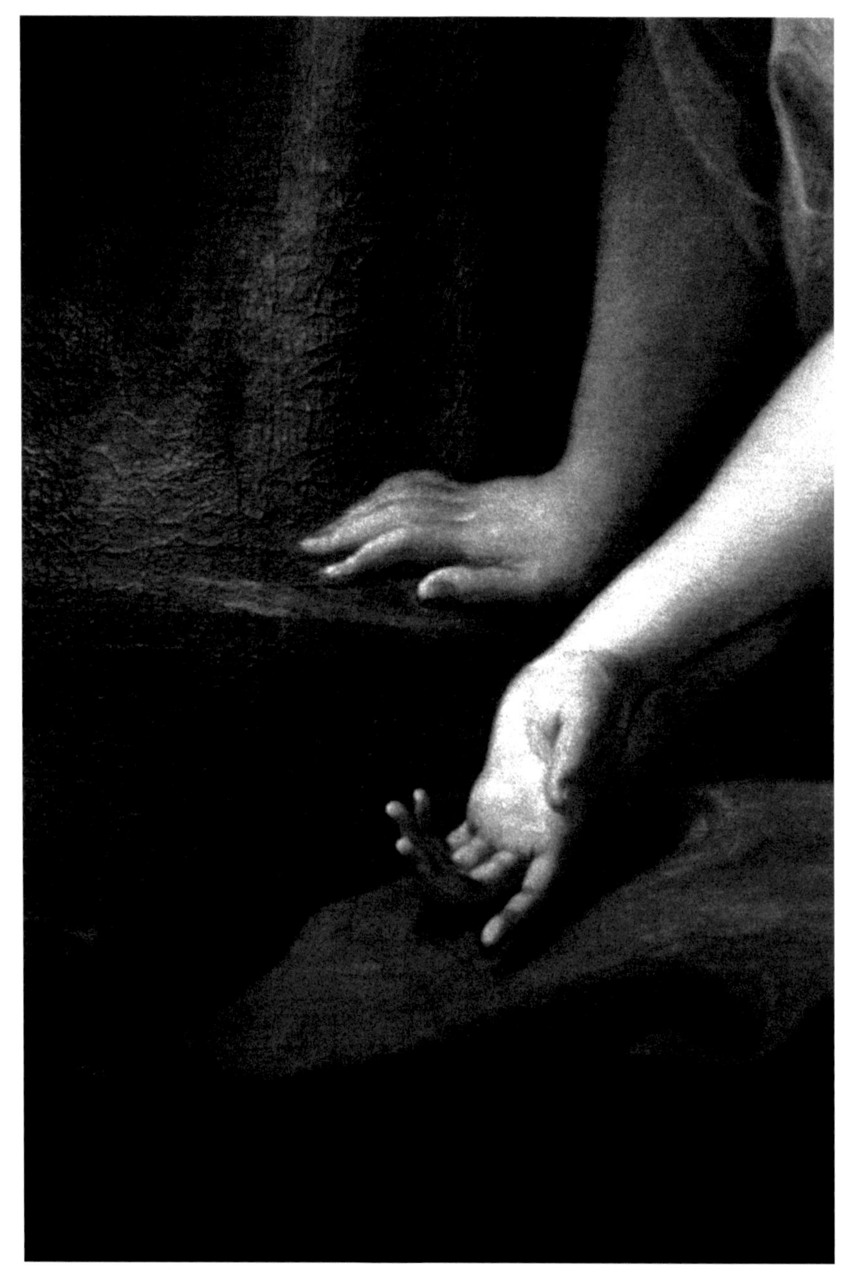

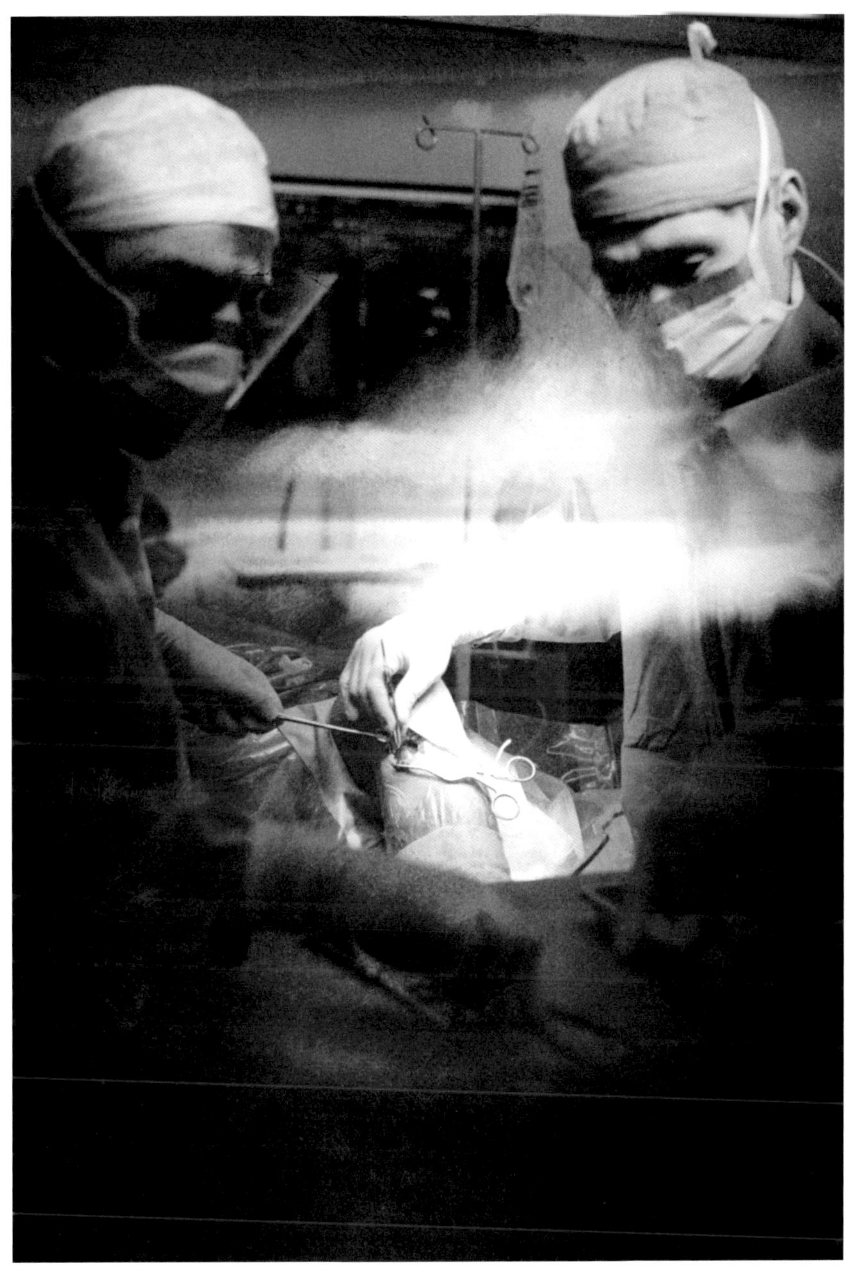

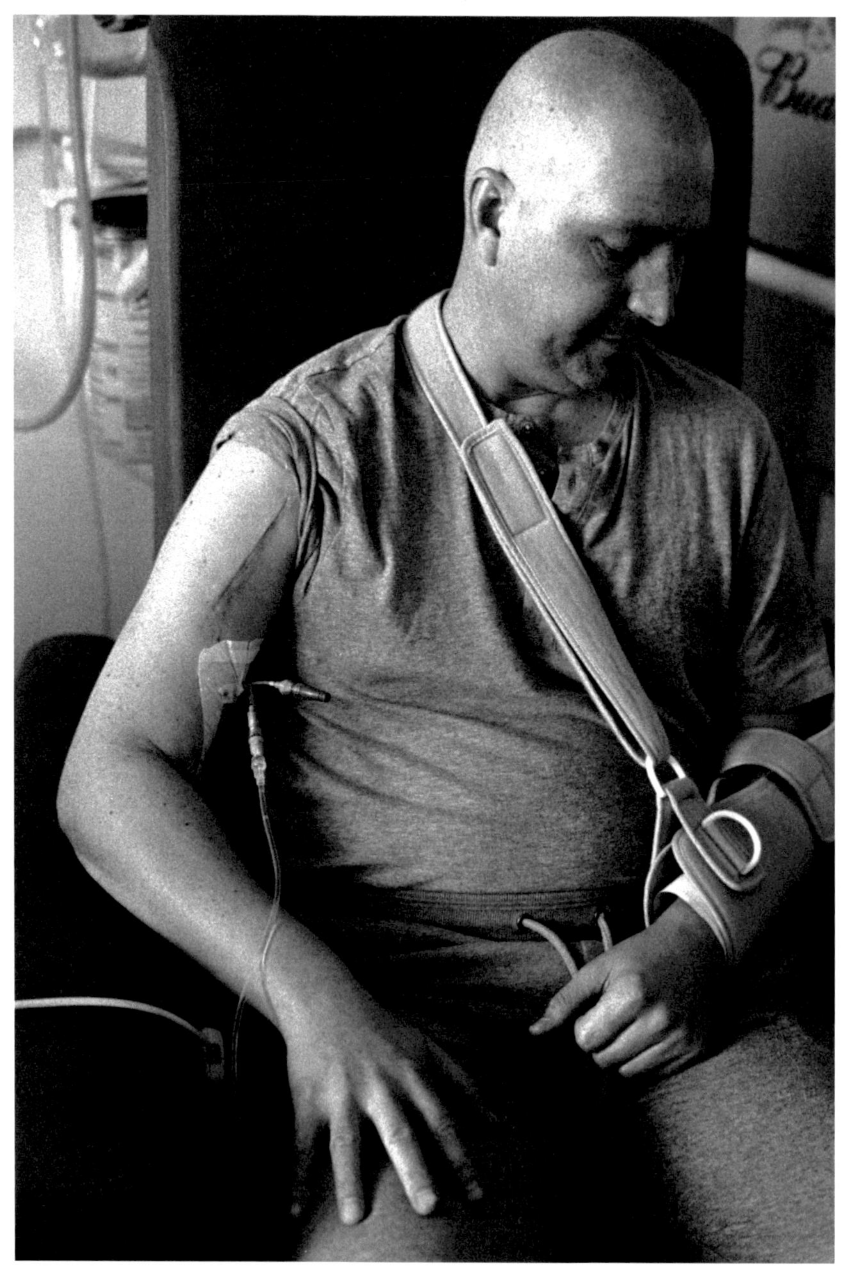

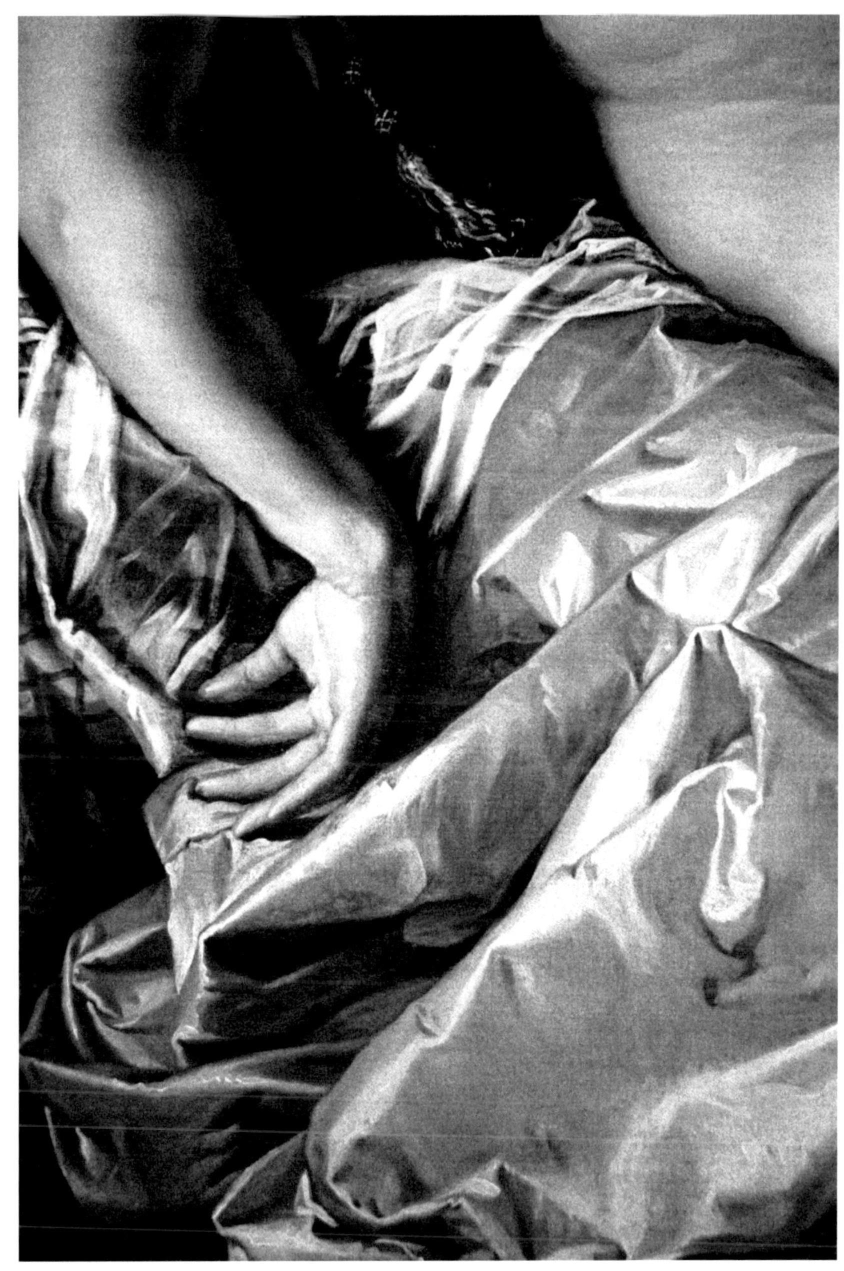

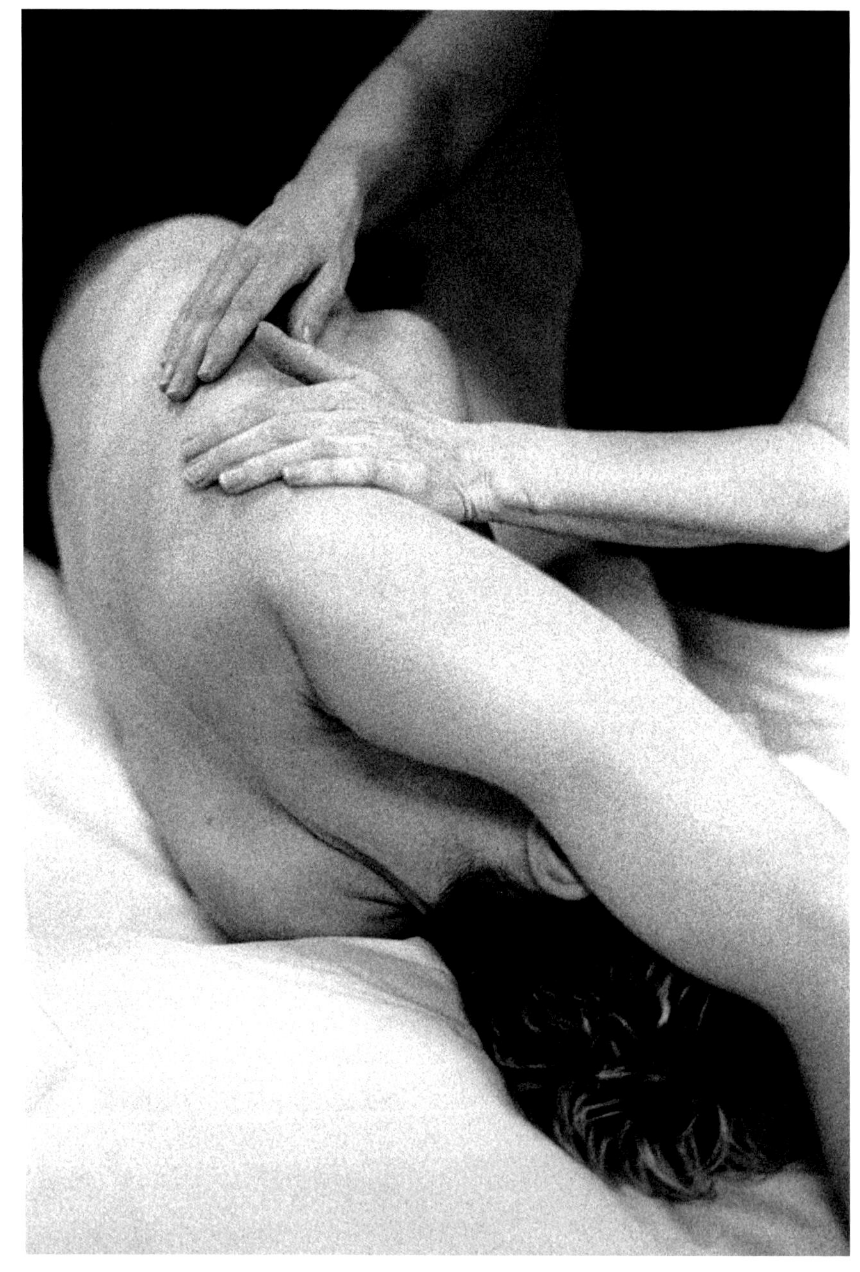

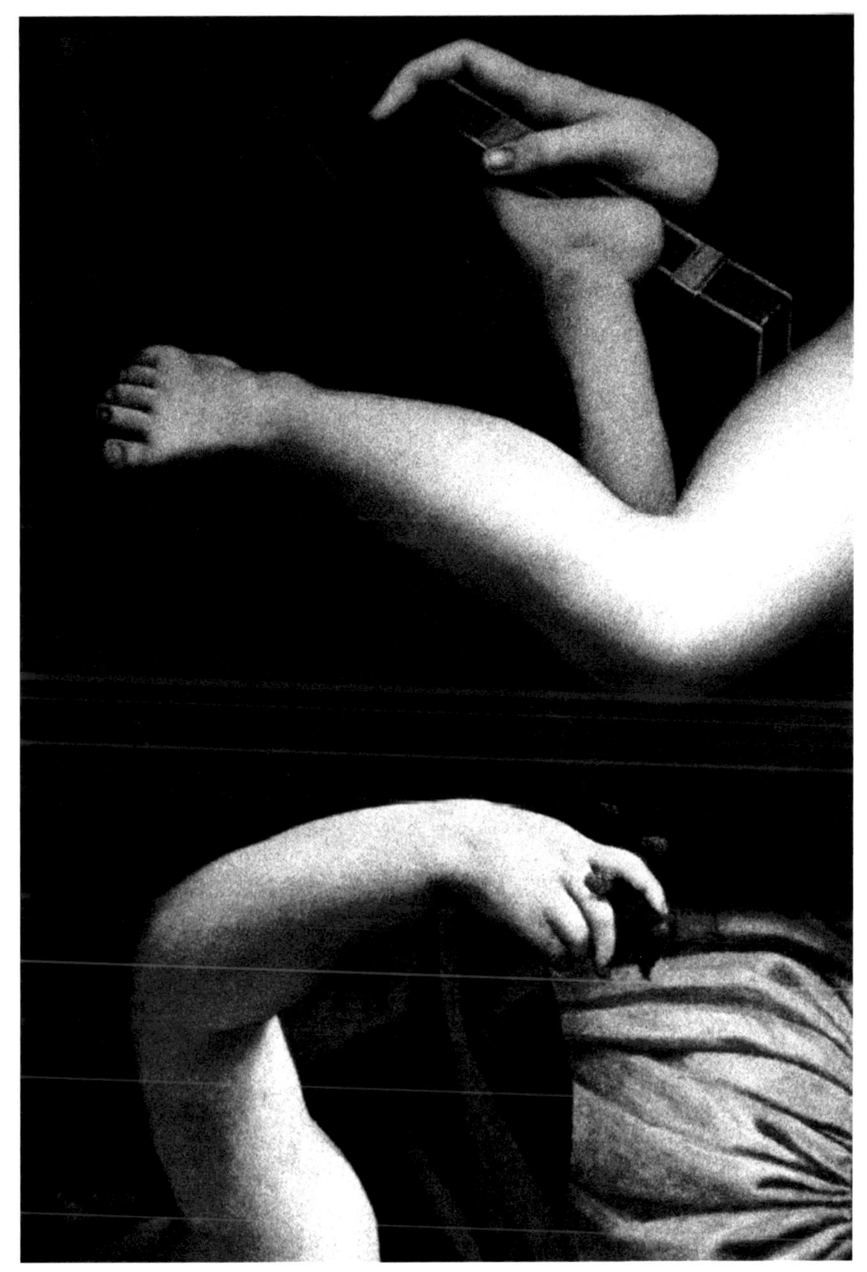

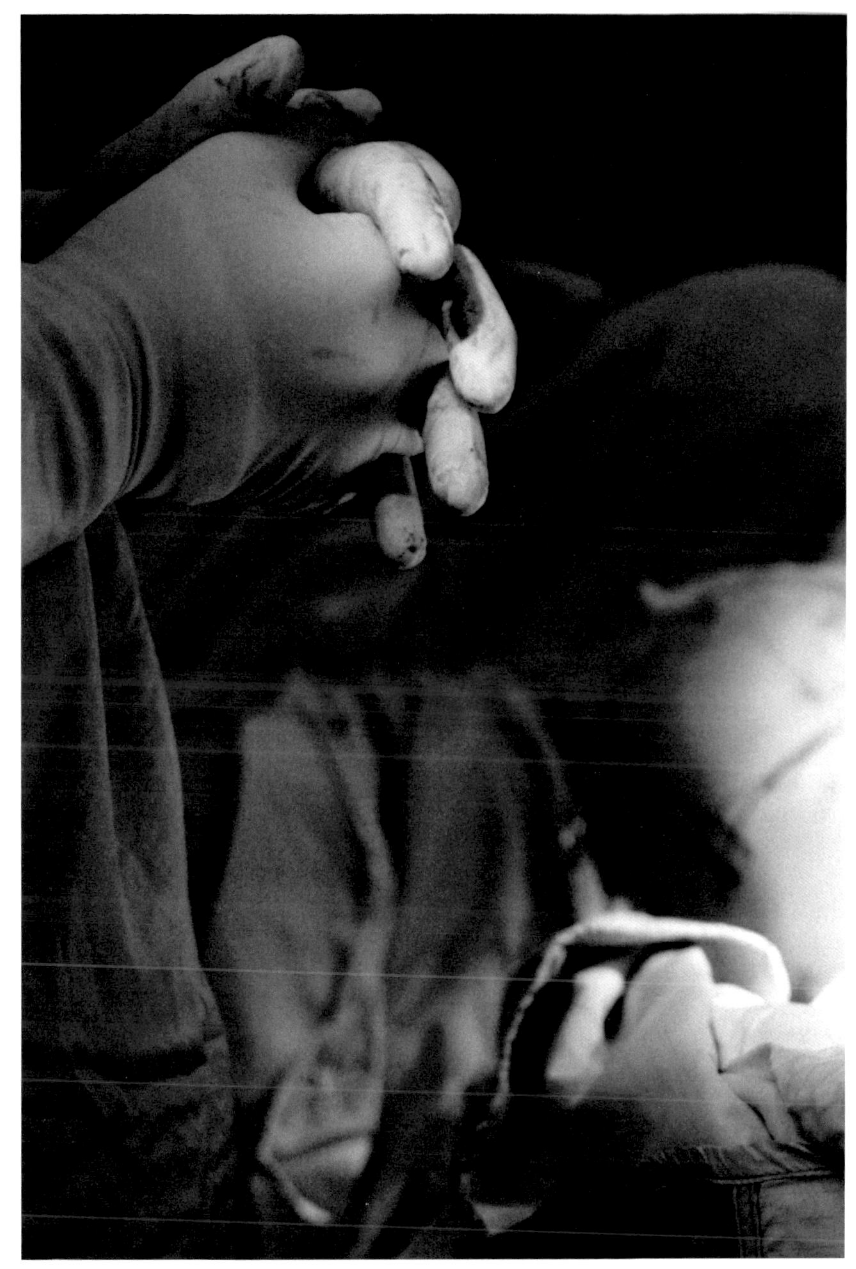

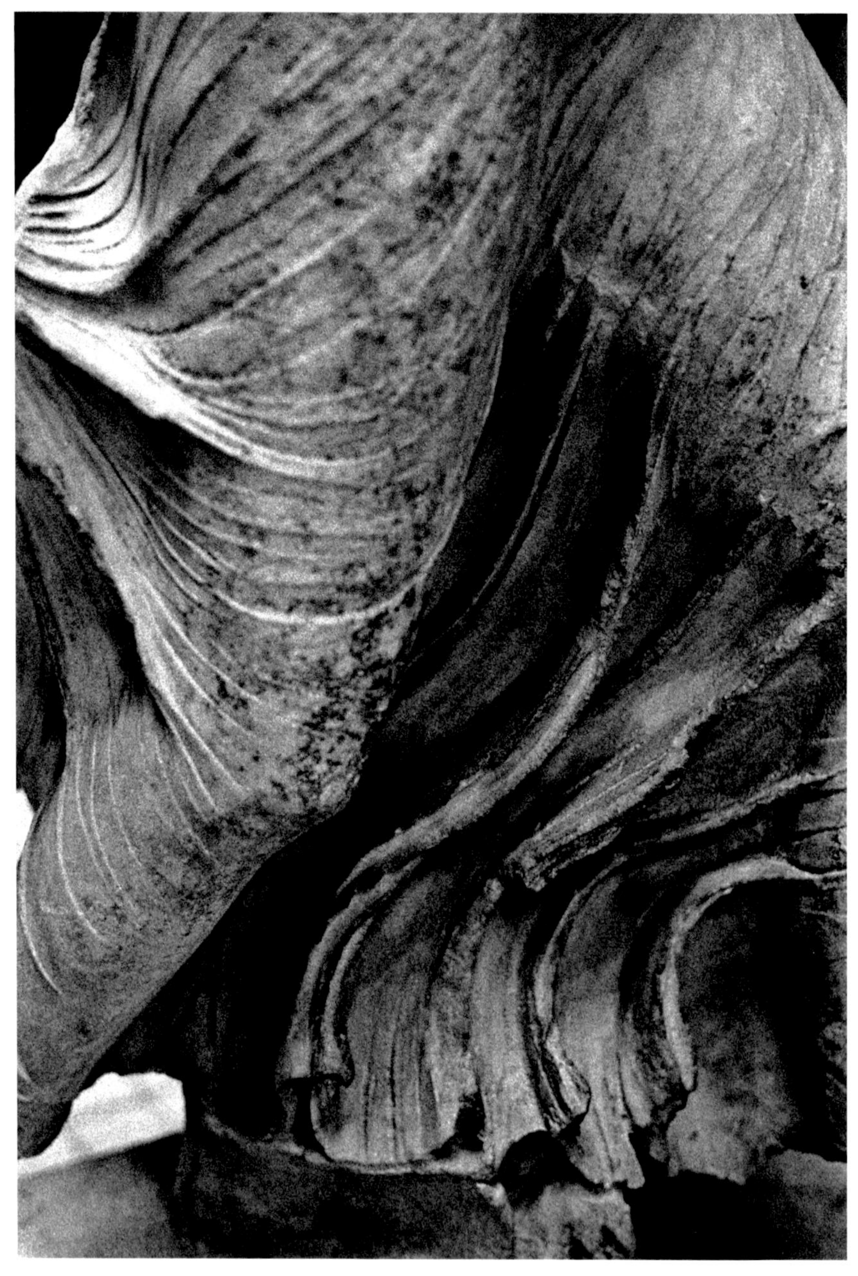

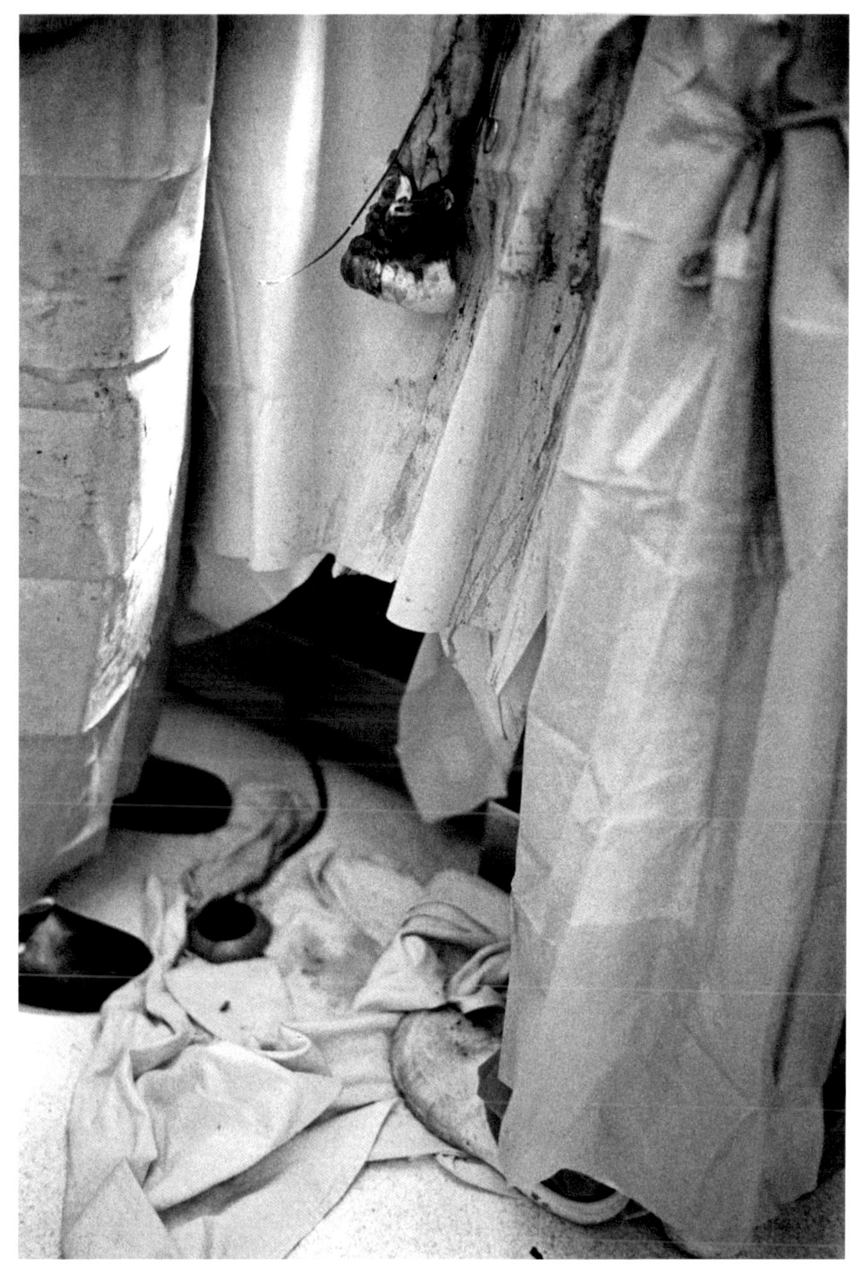

Cut here, says her torso, and here and here and here. Along the thick black lines made by the surgeon earlier that leave her body like a map, so everyone knows the direction of travel and there's no room for doubt.

Still glistening from the ritual washing, with patches placed over her eyes like coins to pay the ferryman, she is ready.

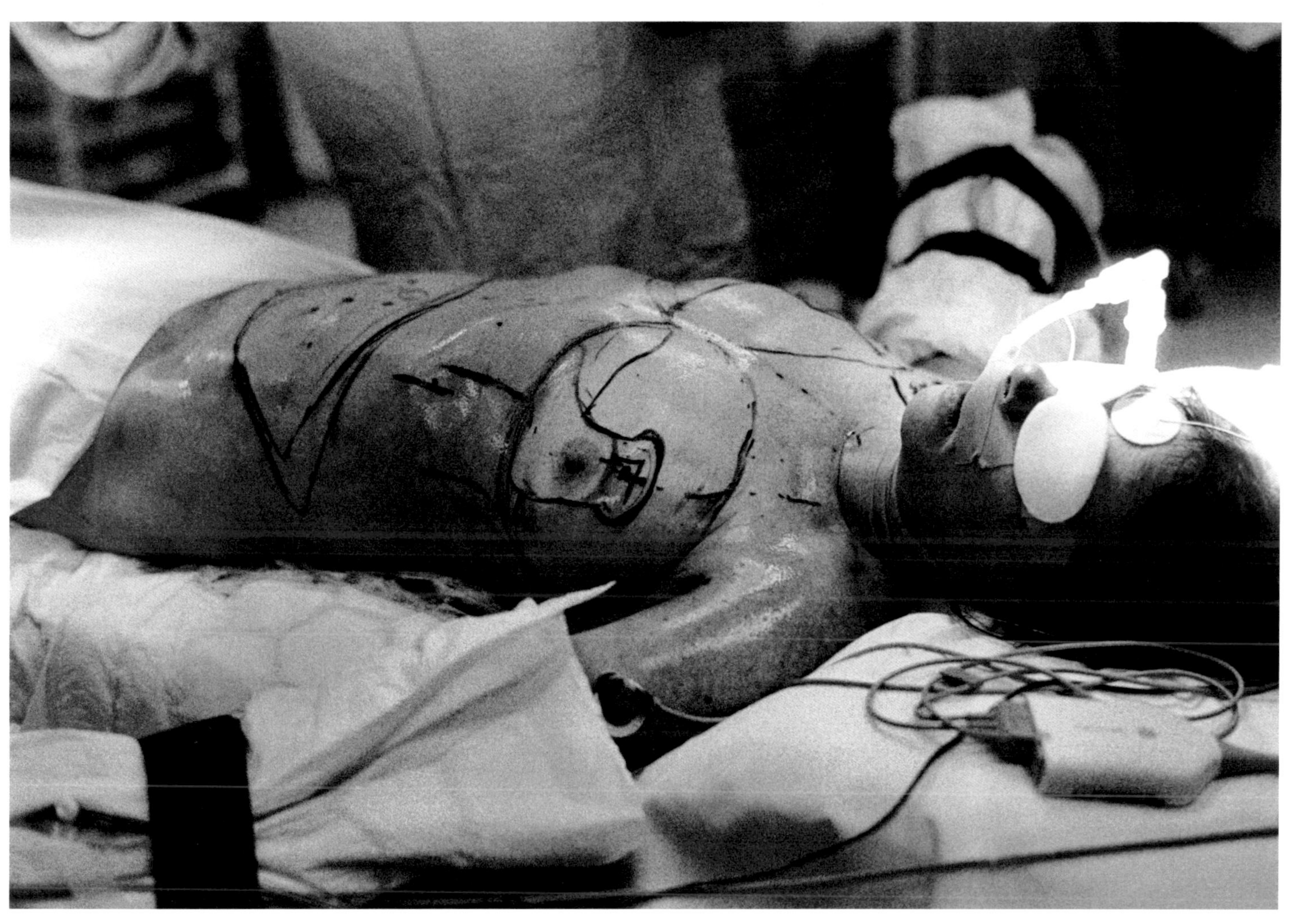

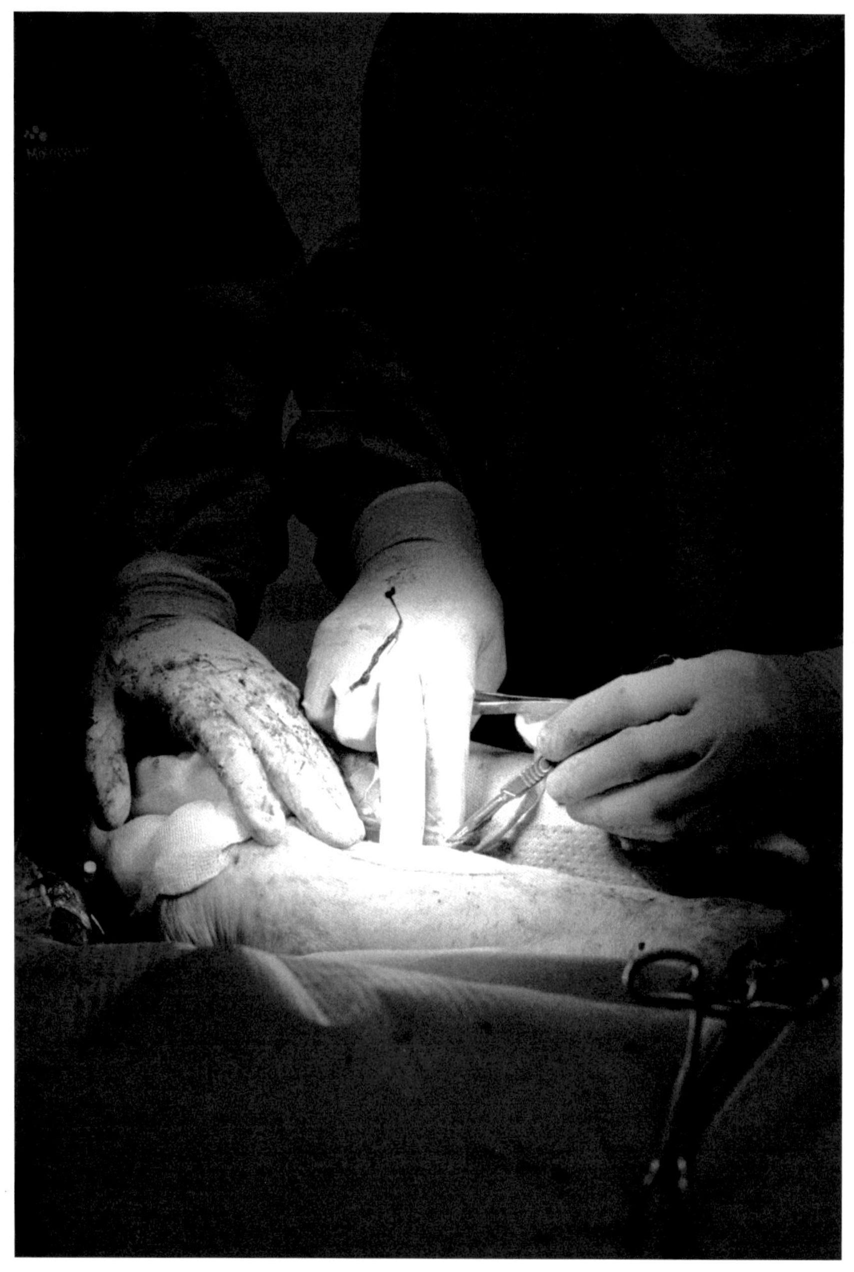

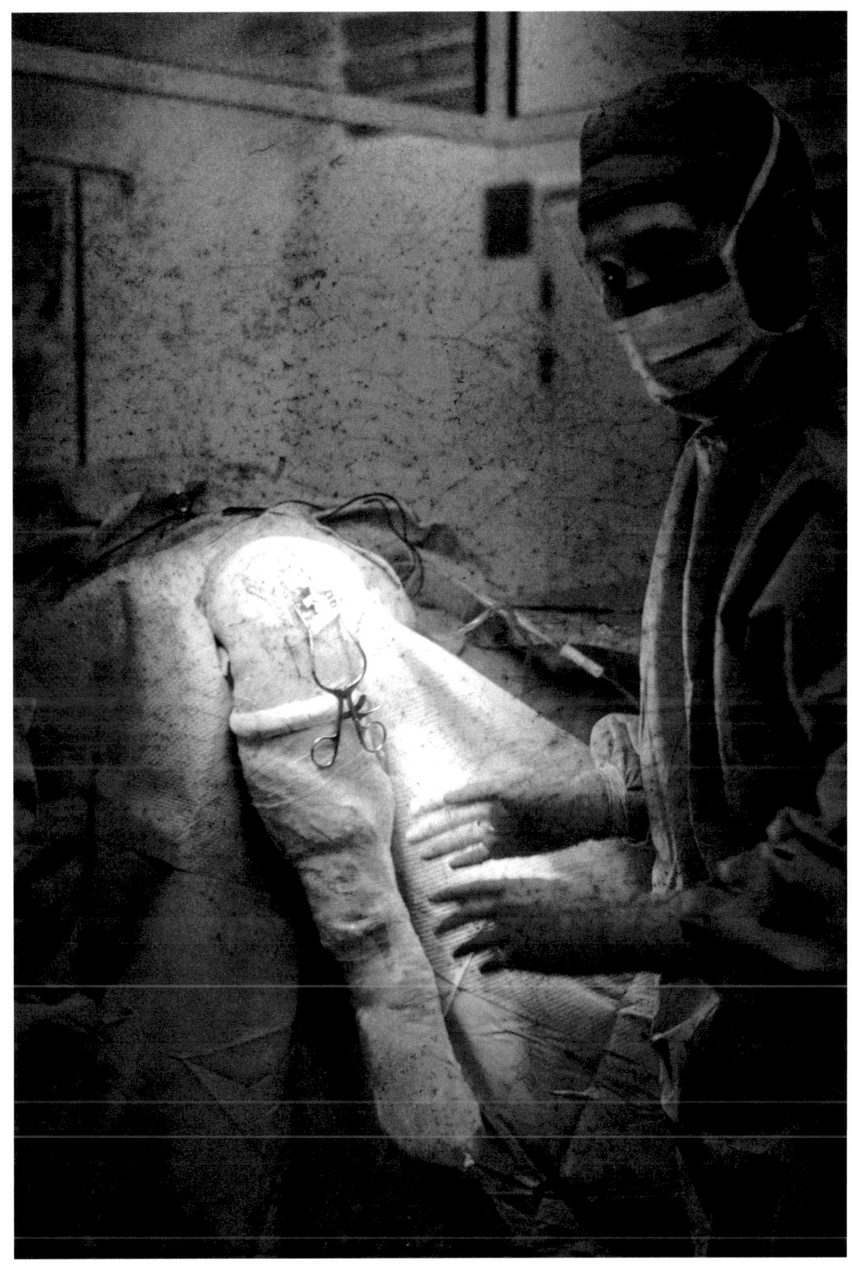

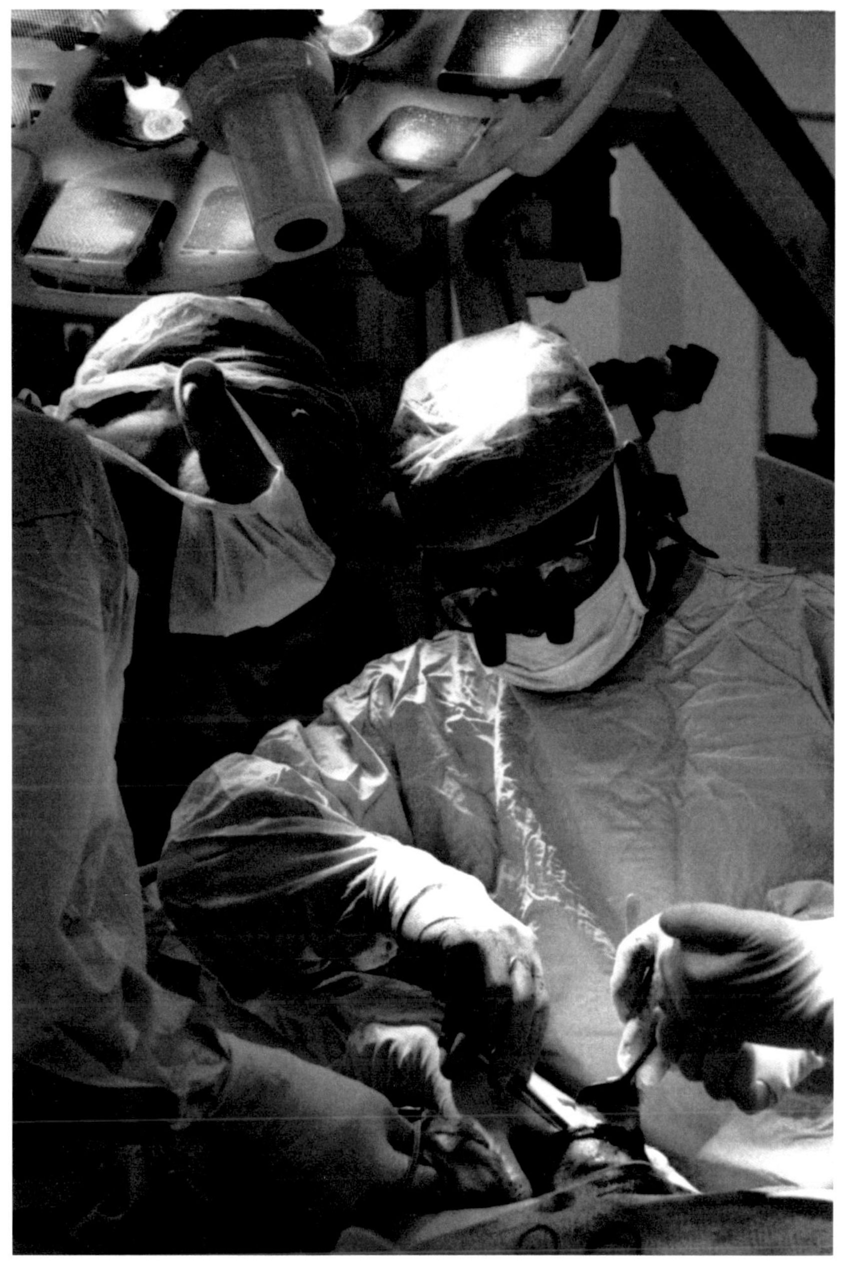

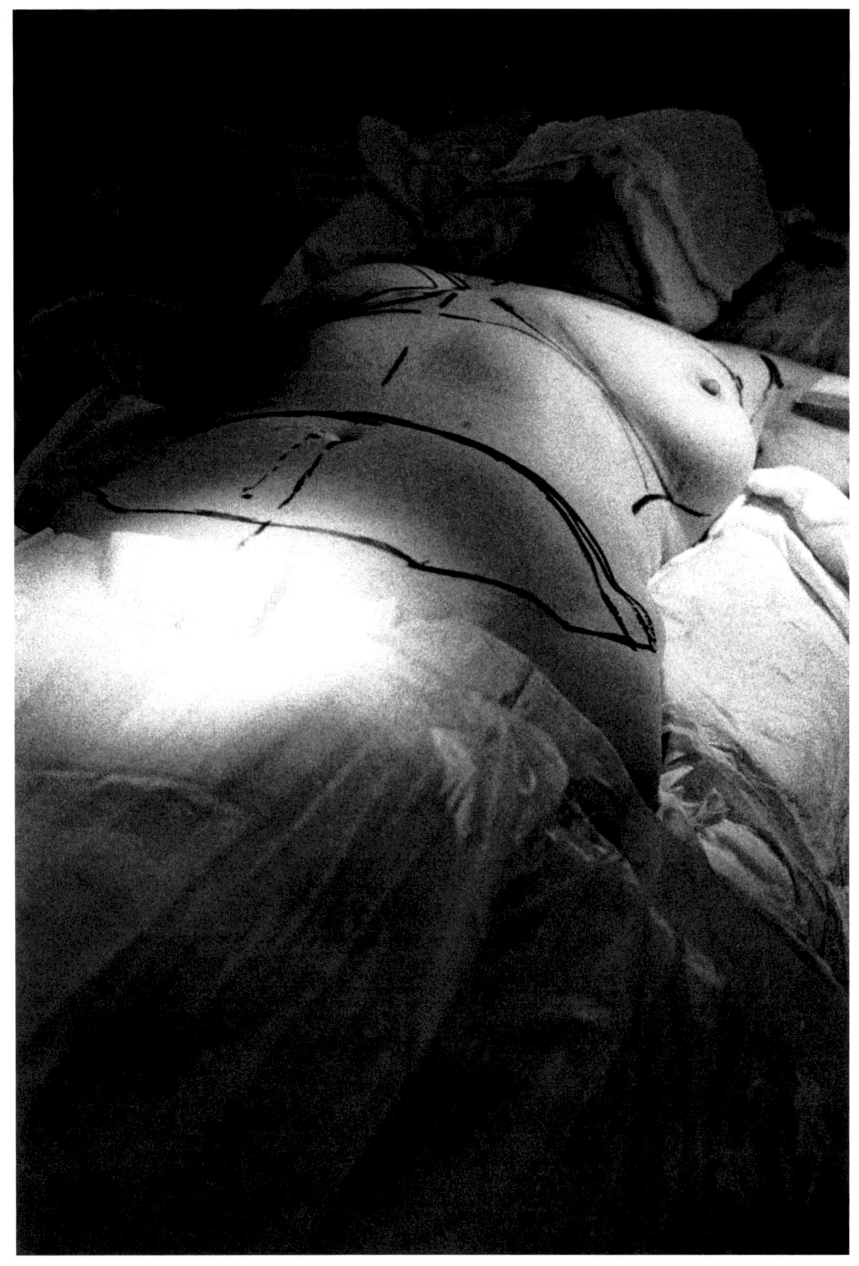

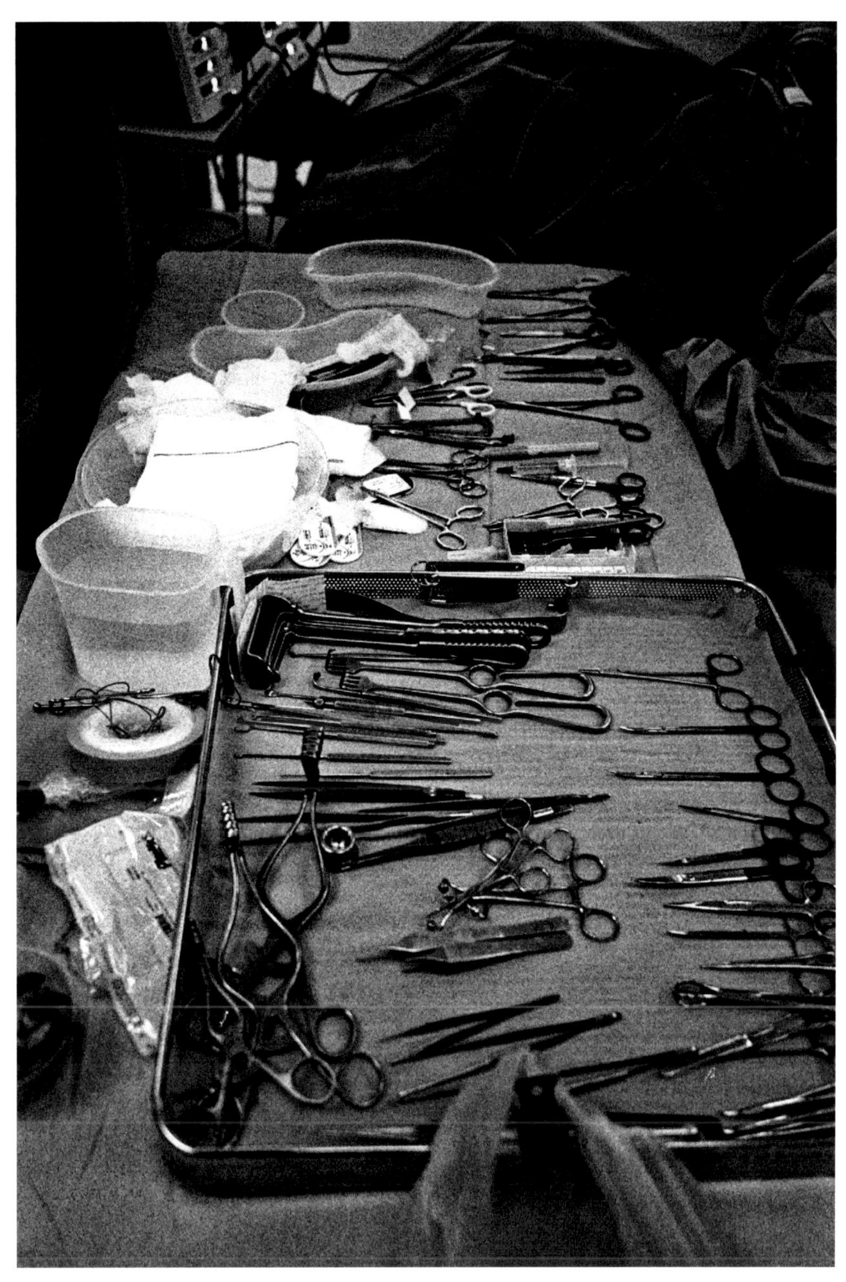

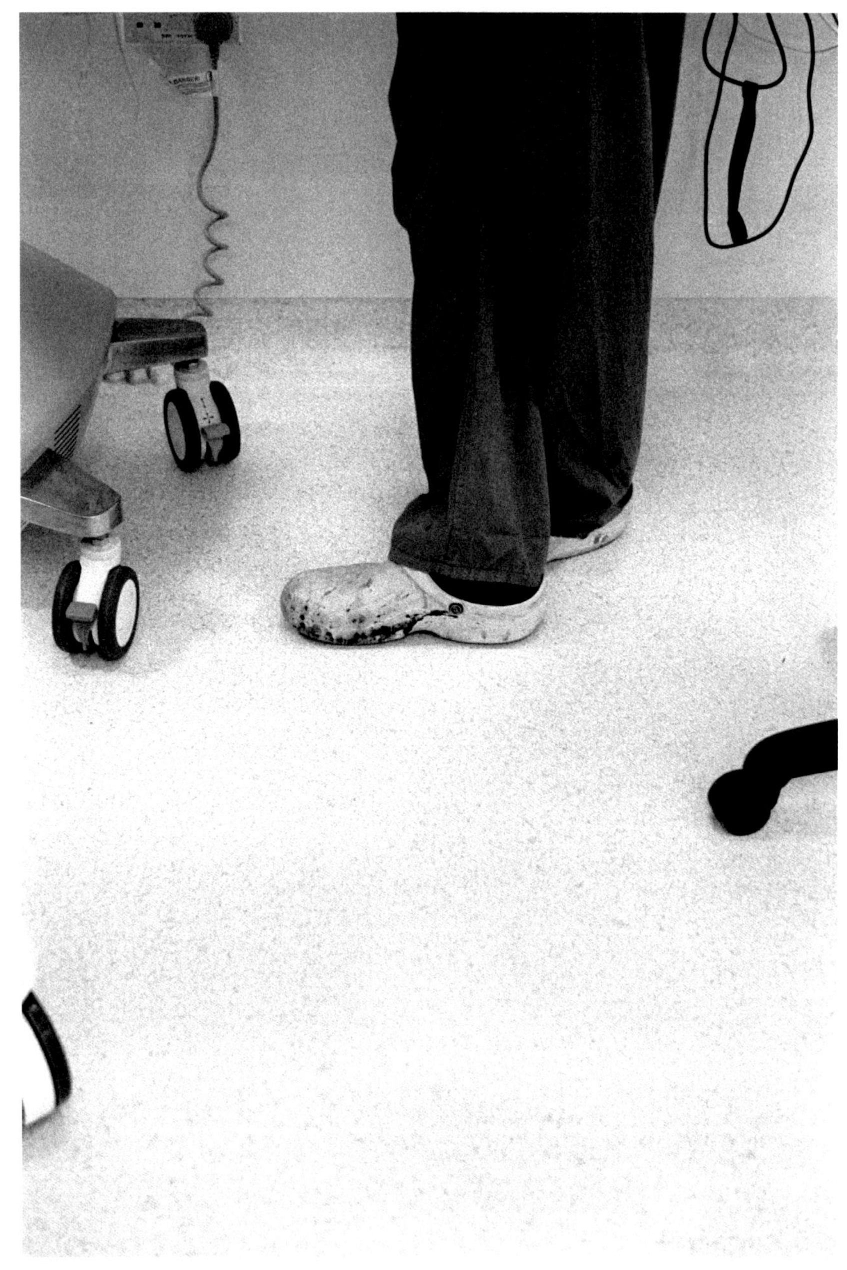

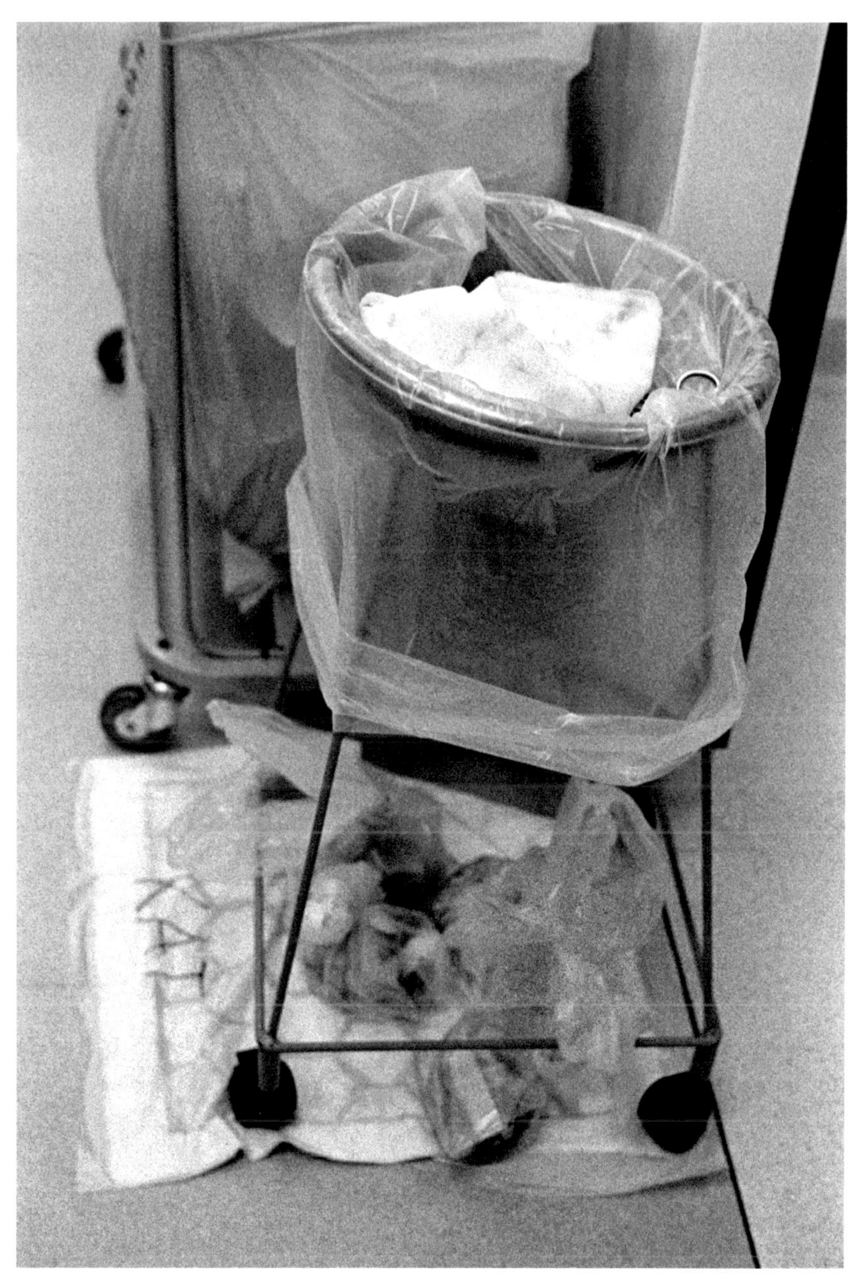
KAT

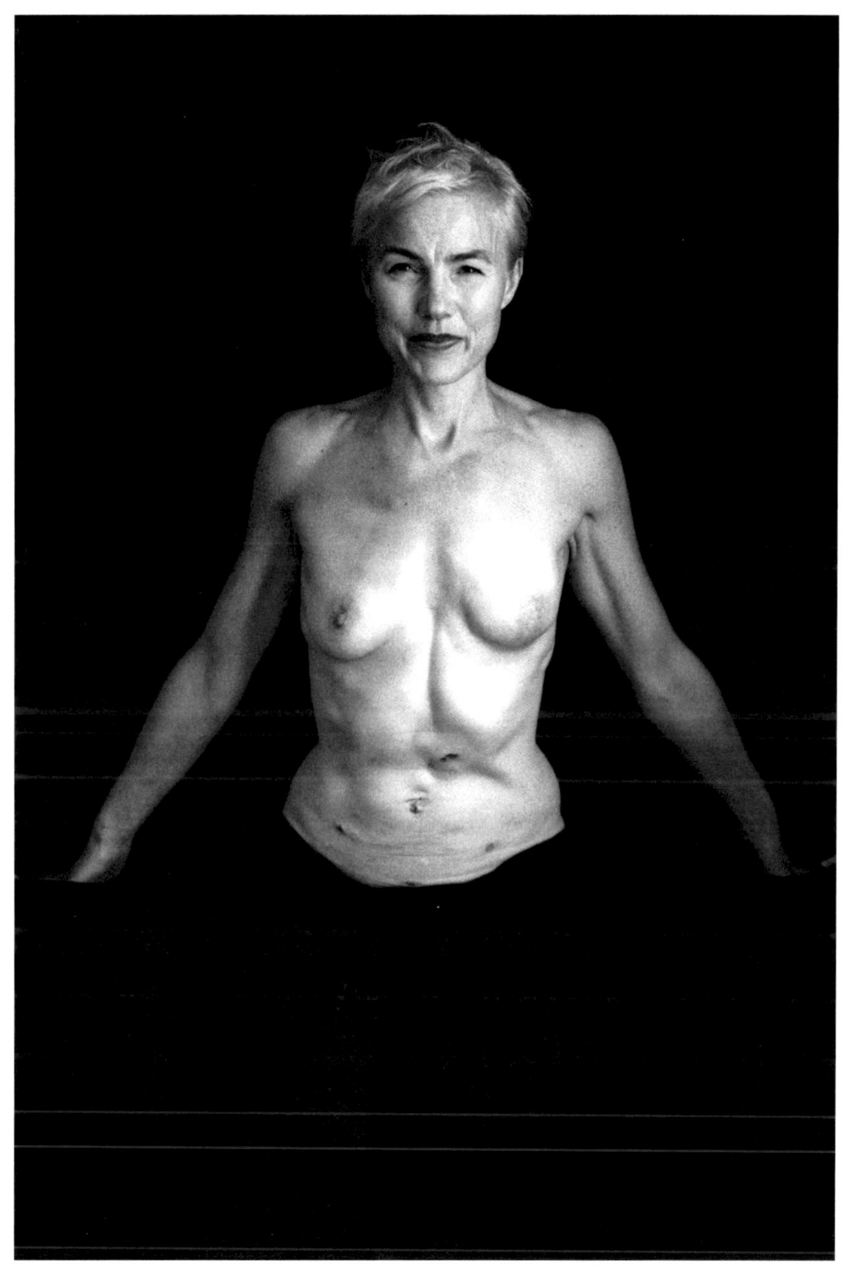

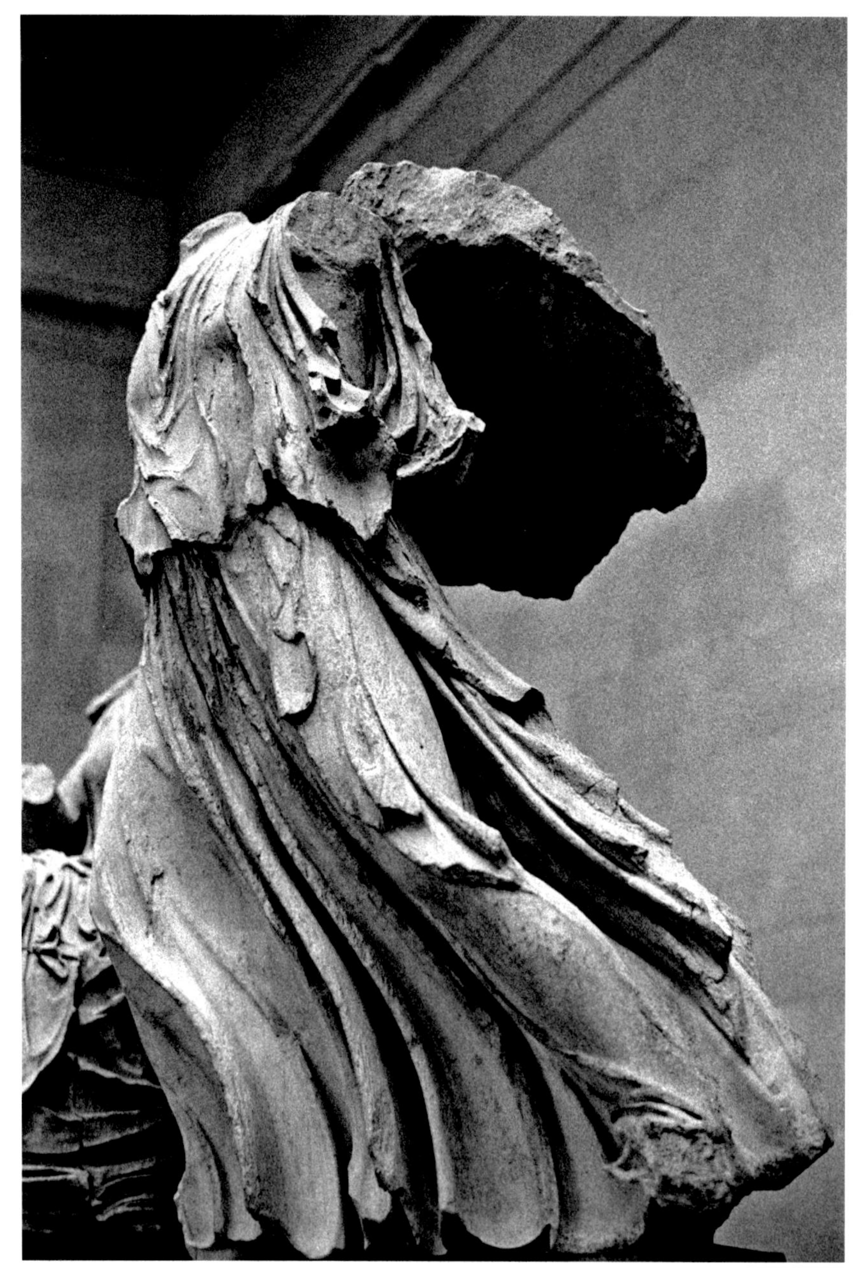

I am indebted to Mr Peter Kalu, Professor Tom Cosker of the Oxford University Hospitals NHS Trust, their teams and their patients; Brenda Kelly, Paddy Summerfield and Patricia Baker-Cassidy; and to Dewi Lewis for his boldness in agreeing to publish this book.

I am grateful to The National Gallery, British Museum and Ashmolean Museum for their kind permission to photograph and publish these details from works in their collections.

Caroline Seymour

First published in the UK in 2024 by
Dewi Lewis Publishing
8 Broomfield Road, Heaton Moor
Stockport SK4 4ND, England

www.dewilewis.com

ISBN: 978-1-916915-02-2

Design: Caroline Seymour and Dewi Lewis
Print: EBS, Verona, Italy